Canine (K9) Tetanus

What Every Dog Owner Needs to Know

Julie Dimmick

This book is a work of independent commentary, research synthesis, and personal interpretation. While it references real events, veterinary research, and publicly available information, all views, conclusions, and interpretations expressed are solely those of the author.

Any references to individuals are made only in the context of publicly available information or lived experience. Any resemblance to private individuals, outside of clearly identifiable public figures or professionals acting in their public capacity, is purely coincidental.

Cover and design layout: Julie Dimmick

First Edition

ISBN: 978-1-7643356-2-1

Published in Australia

ValCoRE Publishing

For permissions, rights, or inquiries, contact: Julie Dimmick author@juliedimmick.com

Printed in Australia.

Disclaimer

This book is a work of lived experience, research synthesis, and educational commentary. It documents one puppy's journey through canine tetanus and draws on published veterinary literature, clinical observations, and the author's personal experience as a dog owner and caregiver.

The author is **not a veterinarian, veterinary nurse, or medically trained professional**. Nothing in this book is intended to diagnose, treat, cure, or prevent disease in animals. References to veterinary conditions, symptoms, treatments, medications, nursing practices, or recovery processes are provided **for general informational and educational purposes only**.

This book does **not** replace professional veterinary care. Readers should never delay, disregard, or substitute veterinary advice based on the content of this book. Any concerns about a dog's health, behaviour, or recovery should always be discussed with a **qualified veterinarian or veterinary specialist**.

While this book references veterinary research, clinical case studies, and commonly accepted treatment principles, outcomes for animals vary widely based on individual circumstances, disease severity, timing of intervention, and professional care. No guarantee of outcome or recovery is expressed or implied.

References to veterinary professionals, clinics, organisations, studies, or institutions are made in good faith for educational context only and are not intended to criticise, diagnose, or attribute fault. Any interpretations offered reflect the author's understanding as a caregiver and advocate, not a clinician.

This book does not represent the views of any veterinary practice, professional body, organisation, or institution with which the author may be or has been affiliated. The material is provided "as is," and readers accept full responsibility for how they interpret and apply its content.

All trademarks, product names, and referenced works remain the property of their respective owners and are used solely for identification, commentary, or educational reference under applicable fair use principles.

For every puppy healing in silence,

and every human who stays.

Acknowledgements

This book exists because of people who showed up with skill, compassion, and steadiness during one of the most confronting chapters of Cher's life.

I wish to acknowledge **Dr Siobhan Doherty**, Cher's everyday veterinarian, whose calm clinical judgement, care, and ongoing oversight were instrumental throughout Cher's illness and recovery. Her willingness to listen, observe closely, and support a long and complex healing process made a profound difference. She held the balance between vigilance and restraint with professionalism and humanity, and Cher's outcome is inseparable from that care.

I also wish to acknowledge **Dr Oscar Huang**, whose deep interest in understanding disease, relentless curiosity, and genuine passion for sharing knowledge with fellow veterinarians exemplifies the kind of medicine that saves lives. It is this commitment to learning, collaboration, and collective advancement that quietly but profoundly keeps animals alive long after the textbooks end.

My thanks also go to **Leona Gielen**, front receptionist at Greencross Biggera Waters, whose kindness, reassurance, and constant support mattered more than she will ever know. In moments of fear and uncertainty, her presence, patience, and genuine care helped carry us through. Compassion at the front desk is not incidental. It shapes the entire experience of care.

I extend my deepest gratitude to **Dr Emily Ireland**, the lead veterinarian who cared for Cher during her time at SASH, where Cher spent her critical period in intensive care. The expertise, vigilance, and decisiveness shown during those ICU days quite literally saved Cher's life. Those moments demanded clarity, endurance, and deep clinical skill, all of which were present when they mattered most.

SASH was where medicine, nursing, and commitment met endurance. I am profoundly grateful to the veterinary and nursing teams who worked tirelessly during Cher's ICU stay, often unseen and under immense pressure, to give her the chance to survive and heal. Their work does not end with stabilisation. It extends through monitoring, restraint, and the long middle that recovery requires.

I also wish to acknowledge **Dr Bantval Anil Prabhu**, an ex-colleague and friend, who I turned to at all hours of the day and night during Cher's illness. Anil kept every conversation honest, grounded, and deeply empathetic. He is a veterinarian who understands the difference between being kind and being real with kindness. He offered clarity without false reassurance, truth without cruelty, and support without ego. His generosity of time, presence, and perspective during the most uncertain moments will be forever valued.

My thanks extend to **Rick from K9 Aquatics at Coomera**, whose expertise and patience were instrumental in Cher's physical recovery. Through carefully managed hydrotherapy, Rick helped guide Cher's muscles and strength back to life step by step, always respecting both her body and her nervous system as they healed. His work exemplified what thoughtful rehabilitation looks like when safety comes before speed.

I am also grateful to **Will and the team at Master of Puppies**, where Cher and Elton attend daycare. As Cher returned to the world, this team worked closely with me to ensure she could enjoy social time while still receiving the rest, regulation, and supervision she needed. Their flexibility, communication, and commitment to Cher's wellbeing supported not just her recovery, but her confidence and joy.

Finally, this book acknowledges the quiet, relentless work of veterinary professionals, rehabilitation specialists, and animal carers everywhere. Their care does not end when the crisis stabilises. It continues through monitoring, restraint, patience, and the long middle of recovery.

Thank you for doing the work that so often goes unseen, and for standing beside animals and the people who love them when it matters most.

Table of Contents

Author's Note *15*

PART I: When Something Isn't Right **17**

Chapter 1 Cher *19*

Chapter 2 The First Signs *31*

Chapter 3 Being Told It Was Nothing *45*

Chapter 4 The Question That Would Not Leave *55*

PART II: The Diagnosis No One Expects **63**

Chapter 5 When the Word Tetanus Appears *67*

Chapter 6 How Tetanus Hides in Plain Sight *77*

Chapter 7 ICU *87*

Chapter 8 What Treatment Really Looks Like *101*

PART III: The Long Middle **111**

Chapter 9 Stabilised Is Not Recovered *119*

Chapter 10 Stillness Is Treatment *129*

Chapter 11 When Appetite Lies *139*

Chapter 12 What the Research Quietly Confirms *151*

Part IV: Returning to Life **161**

Chapter 13 Bringing Her Body Back *167*

Chapter 14 Re-entering the World Safely *177*

Part V: What Every Dog Owner Needs To Know **197**

Chapter 15 Early Warning Signs Owners See First *203*

Chapter 16 What Helps and What Hurts *215*

Chapter 17 When to Insist on Help *225*

Chapter 18 Recovery Timelines and Expectations *233*

Part VI: Why This Story Matters **243**

Chapter 19 For the Puppies Who Come After *249*

Chapter 20 Cher Today *267*

Glossary **279**

ICU Related Terms *281*

Tetanus Related Terms *285*

Growth, Nutrition, and Development During Tetanus Recovery *289*

Veterinary Literature Referenced **291**

About the Author **301**

Author's Note

This book is not a veterinary manual, and I am not a veterinarian or medically trained professional. What follows is not medical advice, nor should it ever replace professional veterinary assessment, diagnosis, or treatment.

This book exists to document lived experience, the kind that unfolds in real time, without certainty, and often without language. It reflects what it is like to notice subtle change, to sit inside uncertainty, to advocate without guarantees, and to carry responsibility long after discharge papers are signed.

Cher's survival was the result of skilled veterinary care, clinical decision-making, and sustained medical support. My role was not to replace that expertise, but to remain present enough to notice when something was not right, persistent enough to return when answers did not settle, and committed enough to carry care forward when recovery moved from hospital to home.

Every dog, every illness, and every outcome is different. Advocacy does not ensure recovery, and vigilance does not prevent loss. What it can do is widen the margin in which understanding, investigation, and care become possible.

This book is offered in service of that margin.

Always seek professional veterinary advice for concerns about your own animal's health or wellbeing.

PART I:

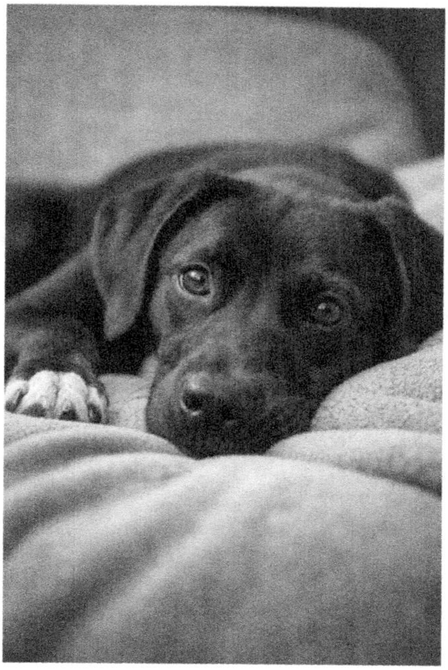

WHEN SOMETHING ISN'T RIGHT

Chapter 1

Cher

Cher was born on 25 August 2025. When she came into my care at seven weeks old, she did not yet know what she was going to become. She moved through the world with the soft misjudgement of a puppy still learning the limits of her own body, falling into paws already too large for her sense of scale. She had no idea she was not a small dog. She had no understanding of the strength that would eventually live in her frame.

What she did have was ease. A natural flow. That unmistakable puppy swagger that comes from a nervous system not yet burdened by caution, memory, or restraint.

Cher came into my life quietly.

No drama. No grand story. Just a small black puppy with too little fur, sore skin, and eyes that looked older than her body. She was still soft with that unmistakable puppy smell, still clumsy, still learning where her legs ended and the world began. She did not arrive whole. Her coat was patchy. Her skin inflamed. Her body fragile in a way you do not always notice at first glance.

From the first night, she cried. Long, searching cries that carried the absence of her mother through the dark. She was crate trained immediately, not as discipline but as a gift. In a home with two large, strong-minded dogs, it mattered that each had a space that was theirs alone. A place to retreat, to pause, to regulate. At the time, it was simply good practice. Later, it would matter far more than I could have known.

Elton was already here.

Elton is steady. Confident. The kind of dog who belongs wherever he stands. Cher followed him everywhere, studying him, copying him, finding safety in his presence. She was careful with novelty. New things were not met with enthusiasm so much as evaluation. She would pause, watch, orient. Unless Elton went first. If Elton moved, Cher followed. If he stood his ground, she took that as information. She was learning the world through him, calibrating herself against his presence.

Under my care, her skin healed. Her coat thickened. Her body filled out. Nourishment came in every sense. Food, rest, touch, consistency. Slowly, deliberately, her coat became lush and shiny. Her body began to reflect the care it was receiving.

Those early weeks were about meeting her needs without urgency or force. Love did the rest.

As she settled, her nervous system softened. She learned how to pause, how to play and then rest. Safety was simple. It was me. It was Elton. Food arrived consistently. Boundaries were clear. Trust followed.

She arrived with sharp resource guarding around food, intense for such a young puppy. With steady home-based training, and with Elton modelling calm and patience, that shifted. Eventually they ate from the same bowl. Food became abundant rather than contested. She let me place my hand in her bowl while she ate. She followed me without hesitation from room to room.

Cher was adorable in a way that was almost disarming. Not delicate. Not ornamental. Adorable in motion. In expression. In the way her oversized paws slapped the floor slightly out of sync with the rest of her body. Her ears never quite decided what they wanted to do. One would lift in curiosity while the other lagged behind. Her eyes held that earnest intensity puppies have when they are trying very hard to understand what is expected of them.

She wanted to get it right.

From the beginning, we worked on foundations. Not tricks. Not performance. Foundations. Sit meant pause. Wait meant regulate. Down meant soften the body. Release meant permission. These were not commands so much as language. She learned quickly, not because she was pushed, but because she was attentive. She watched faces. She watched hands. She read tone before she processed words.

During dinner routines, both dogs were required to lie down and hold position until released. Elton would drop and wait with the patience of an old soul. Cher would drop, give a small puppy yap of protest, spring up in excitement, then drop again. Over and over. It was not defiance. It was enthusiasm wrestling with self-control. Eventually the pause between impulse and action grew longer. That is how regulation is built. Not by force, but by repetition and calm correction.
She loved to learn.

When I clipped the lead on for early neighbourhood walks, she would prance beside me for the first few metres, then suddenly remember she was a puppy and leap sideways at a leaf, a shadow, a sound. Each redirection was gentle. Each return to heel celebrated. Behaviour was not about dominance. It was about clarity. The world made more sense to her when expectations were consistent.

In the backyard, she invented games. A stick became treasure. A patch of grass became a hiding place. A single tennis ball was enough to convince her that life could not possibly get better than this. She would sprint in tight, clumsy circles, then collapse dramatically onto her side as though exhausted beyond repair, only to spring up seconds later when Elton moved.

With Elton, she was bold. She would launch herself at him in full body commitment, paws wide, jaw open in exaggerated puppy ferocity. He absorbed her chaos with steady patience. If she became too insistent, he corrected her with a look or a stillness that needed no sound. She learned boundaries not through fear, but through clarity. That is how dogs teach one another.

She adored human contact just as much. When tired, she folded herself into impossible shapes at my feet, chin resting on my shoe as though proximity alone regulated her. If I moved rooms, she followed. If I sat down, she leaned. Physical closeness was reassurance.

She carried herself with a curious contradiction. Protective long before her body had earned the right to be. If she perceived a threat, she would position herself between me and whatever she had decided required intervention, chest out, baby bark at the ready. Later that same day, she would roll onto her back for a belly rub, utterly surrendered.

There was something almost comedic about her determination. If a command required three attempts, she would give four. If a game required speed, she offered exuberance instead. Her mischief was exploratory rather than destructive. A few shallow holes in the garden marked her archaeological curiosity. Nothing more.

Her growth felt visible week to week. Muscle forming under fur. Coordination improving. Confidence stabilising. She began attending doggy daycare, carefully supervised at first. Hydrotherapy sessions strengthened her body while building resilience. Playdates expanded her social vocabulary. Each new environment was introduced slowly. Evaluated. Then embraced.

She was learning how to be a good dog.

Not compliant. Not suppressed. Regulated. Curious. Social. Clear on boundaries. Secure in attachment. That foundation matters more than people realise. It creates a baseline. And baseline is everything when something shifts.

There were things I never worried about. Her appetite. Her thirst. Her movement.

She ate enthusiastically, matching Elton bowl for bowl and finishing his leftovers without apology. Her movement was free and fluid. Her eyes were soft and open. Her breathing was easy, punctuated only by the deep snores of a growing puppy asleep at night. She slept soundly. She played hard. Nothing about her suggested fragility.

That is the part people like to hear. What they do not see is how quickly everything can unravel.

It started with her eyes. Not redness. Not discharge. Just something off. They did not rest the way they should. They seemed tense, watchful even when she was tired. Her face looked different in subtle ways that are almost impossible to describe unless you know a dog well enough to notice when their expressions shift.

I was told it was conjunctivitis. Then chemosis. Then irritation. Nothing serious. Puppies get things. Puppies grow through things.

But I knew something was not right. Not dramatically wrong. Not emergency obvious. Just wrong in the way that tightens your stomach even when logic tells you to relax.

Her movements became careful. Her muscles never seemed to fully let go. Then came the snorting. Brief at first. Easy to dismiss. Puppies make noises. Dogs snort. But this was not normal.

Over days, not hours, her body began to change. Her muscles tightened. Her face stiffened. Her movements became deliberate, as though the world suddenly required more effort. Rest did not restore her. Excitement drained her quickly. She was still eating. Still wagging. Still my puppy. But she was not relaxing.

Illness does not always announce itself. Sometimes it whispers.

I went back to the vet. Then again. And again. Each time the answers were reasonable. Logical. Comforting. None of them explained why my puppy's body seemed to be forgetting how to soften.

By the time the word tetanus was finally spoken, Cher's nervous system was already under siege.

Tetanus does not arrive like an infection you can see. It arrives as tension. As vigilance without rest. As muscles that will not let go. As a body locked in permanent readiness.

Cher was hospitalised. Sedated. Monitored. Fed carefully. Moved gently. Protected from noise, light, excitement, from everything a growing puppy should have been enjoying.

Recovery did not look like healing. It looked like stillness.

It looked like crate rest when she wanted to play. It looked like saying no when she tried to bounce back too quickly. It looked like watching her breathe, swallow, blink, over and over, learning her patterns the way nurses do in intensive care.

Some days she improved. Some days she went backwards. There were moments when her body betrayed her again. Vomiting from stimulation. Muscle tension triggered by excitement. Neurological reminders that the toxin had not finished its work.

This is the part of tetanus most people never see. What I have come to call the long middle. The bacteria can be treated. The wound, if one is even found, can be cleaned. But the toxin binds to the nervous system and refuses to be rushed. Recovery becomes vigilant waiting. Every decision matters.
Cher did not need heroics.

She needed protection.
She needed time.
She needed someone willing to trust what they were seeing, even when improvement did not look like progress.

Cher lived.

She healed slowly. Unevenly. Patiently. She is now a solid, strong girl, still carrying the memory of tetanus in her nervous system, but no longer living from it. Each day her baseline moves further toward health.

This book begins with Cher because her story is not rare. It is simply rarely told in full.

What saves them is not a miracle drug.
It is recognition. Persistence. And the quiet refusal to accept "she's fine" when fine does not feel true.

Once tetanus takes hold, love looks a lot like restraint.

Chapter 2

The First Signs

The first signs of tetanus do not look like tetanus. They do not arrive as crisis, and they do not announce themselves with urgency or spectacle. They do not force decisions or interrupt life in a way that demands immediate action. Instead, they slip quietly into the ordinary rhythm of days, wearing the disguise of normal variation. They arrive softly, settle comfortably into routine, and wait to be explained away.

They present as small things, the kind that are noticed briefly and then rationalised. They register just long enough to trigger a passing thought before being filed under puppy behaviour, development, or nothing to worry about. They feel slightly off, but not wrong enough to slow momentum or halt the day. This is how tetanus survives unseen, by embedding itself within the ordinary and borrowing the credibility of normality.

Looking back, I am no longer certain that what I noticed first was actually the beginning. That uncertainty is one of the cruellest features of this illness. Tetanus does not reveal its entry point or provide a clean starting line. Instead, it creates a blur in which early signs overlap so convincingly with everyday life that certainty only arrives later, when hindsight sharpens everything and the question becomes not what was missed, but how it managed to hide for so long.

What I remember noticing first were her eyes, not because they looked injured or inflamed, but because something about them did not belong in a resting puppy. There was no redness, no discharge, and no swelling that demanded concern. What caught my attention was harder to name. Her eyes did not soften easily or drift into rest. Even when her body appeared tired, her gaze remained alert, as though her nervous system could not complete the transition from activation to release.

At first, this presented as something almost imperceptible. There was a fleeting sense that her eyes were too focused and too present. They followed movement with a vigilance that did not fade with familiarity, and even in quiet moments, when a puppy should dissolve into ease, there was a watchfulness that lingered. It was subtle enough to doubt, but persistent enough to return to awareness.

Over time, there were moments when her eyes rolled back more than they should have. This was not dramatic and not constant, but it occurred often enough to be noticed. When she looked upward, when she became fatigued, or when stimulation accumulated, the whites of her eyes appeared briefly and then remained visible longer than expected. At times, her third eyelid surfaced partway, covering the eye even though she was awake, responsive, and otherwise calm. What I was seeing did not resemble irritation, injury, or infection in any of the familiar ways those conditions usually present. Instead, it became increasingly apparent that muscular control itself was behaving differently than it should have been, as though the systems responsible for releasing tension were no longer functioning as expected.

The muscles around her eyes appeared unable to fully release. Even at rest, they remained subtly engaged, holding tension where there should have been softness. This was the kind of change that is easy to miss and even easier to rationalise. Puppies develop unevenly. Puppies rub their faces. Eye irritation is common. Growth comes in bursts. Every one of those explanations was reasonable, and every one of them made sense, except that this change did not resolve.

Days passed and then more days, and the tension remained. It did not escalate dramatically, but it did not disappear either. It simply stayed, constant and quiet, present without demanding explanation. Alongside the changes in her eyes came another shift so ordinary that it barely registered at first. Cher began to drink more water, not excessively or urgently, but more often. She returned to the bowl repeatedly, lingered there longer, and needed it refilled more frequently than before.

On its own, this meant very little. Puppies drink more as they grow. Active dogs drink more. Warm weather increases thirst. None of this raised alarm. What made it significant in hindsight was its consistency. This was not a single warm day or a short phase. It was a steady pattern that appeared alongside the other changes, quietly reinforcing something that had not yet fully taken shape.

Physiologically, it made sense. A body under constant muscular tension expends more energy. Muscles that cannot fully relax generate heat, consume resources, and increase the need for hydration long before anything overt appears. At the time, however, it was simply another detail observed and set aside, not dramatic enough to escalate and not specific enough to name.

As days passed, the changes spread across her face. There was a frown that was not an expression of emotion but a structural shift. Her forehead appeared to draw inward, the skin across her brow tightening instead of smoothing out. Where there should have been mobility and softness, there was contraction. Her ears told the same story. They did not relax when she rested. They sat closer together at the top of her head, held there not by curiosity or alertness, but by effort. They did not flick easily in response to sound, remaining fixed as though the muscles responsible for movement were reluctant to let go.

Gradually, her face began to look different, not thin from weight loss and not sick in the way illness is usually recognised, but stripped of ease. The openness that gives a puppy's face its softness began to retreat. The muscles around her eyes, muzzle, and forehead appeared engaged simultaneously, as though her face were bracing against something unseen. This kind of change is difficult to describe unless you know a dog's face intimately and live closely enough with them to recognise when their baseline shifts. It was subtle, easy to doubt, and hard to articulate, but once seen, it could not be unseen.

As time went on, the tension deepened. The muscles around her muzzle and forehead tightened further, and her expression took on a quality of restraint rather than pain or fear. Throughout this period, she remained gentle, responsive, and engaged, continuing to eat well and interact with the world in ways that outwardly aligned with what a young puppy should look like as she moved through her days. From the outside, there was little that would immediately signal distress or illness to someone who did not know her well, yet beneath that familiarity her body was not relaxing in the way it should have been.

When she lay down, there was no sense of her body melting into rest, and when she slept, her muscles remained partially engaged rather than releasing fully. Even in moments that should have allowed recovery, her nervous system appeared to hover in a state of readiness it could not exit, holding tension continuously instead of cycling between activation and ease. I often found myself wondering what that must have felt like for a young puppy still discovering her own body, living inside muscles that would not soften, and experiencing the world through a system that could not fully stand down.

Then a sound began to appear, a strange snort that was brief and intermittent and easy to dismiss. Dogs make noises, and puppies experiment with their airways and breath. It did not sound dangerous or look dramatic or painful, but it persisted. Not frequently enough to provoke panic and not violently enough to demand emergency care, but often enough to settle into awareness and add weight to the growing sense that her body was doing more work than it should have been.

Over days rather than hours, her movement began to change. She became careful and deliberate, not weak and not clumsy, but precise. Each step appeared considered, and each transition required effort. Play tired her more quickly than expected, and excitement drained her faster than her age or conditioning could explain, as though her system were expending energy it could not easily recover. She still wagged her tail, followed Elton everywhere, and engaged with the world as a puppy should, but beneath that familiarity, her body was labouring.

This is how tetanus enters a household, quietly and without spectacle. There is often no obvious wound or injury that marks a clear beginning. Infection can occur through tiny breaks in the skin, healing scratches, or punctures that close before they are noticed, and sometimes there is nothing visible at all.

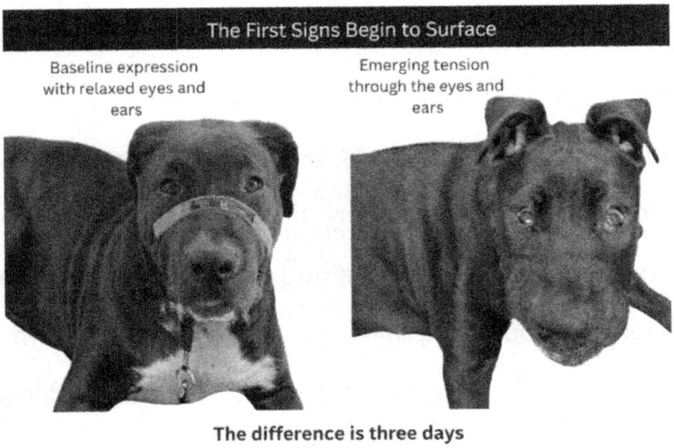

This is Cher, photographed three days apart, during the earliest phase of tetanus, when visible changes in the eyes and ears appeared before the condition was clearly identifiable.

By the time tetanus is suspected, the disease has often already progressed beyond the point where a single intervention can neatly reverse what has begun. This is one of the most confronting realities of the illness. Tetanus does not pause for recognition or wait for clarity to emerge. By the time symptoms gather enough weight to trigger serious concern, the toxin has often already travelled along the nervous system, interfering with the signalling that governs muscle relaxation and autonomic control. What appears to be the beginning, when viewed later, is frequently already well underway.

This delay is not the result of carelessness or a lack of concern. It is structural to the disease itself. Tetanus advances quietly, without dramatic markers that usually signal urgency. There is rarely a moment when everything suddenly aligns and demands immediate action. Instead, there is a slow accumulation of small deviations, each plausible on its own and easily absorbed into ordinary life. By the time those deviations form a coherent picture, the body has often been working against the toxin for longer than anyone realised.

Cher's early signs were not dismissed or ignored. They were noticed, questioned, and returned to for reassessment. They were examined in light of new observations and weighed carefully against what was known at the time. Each decision was made with care and grounded in professional judgement and the information available in that moment, yet those signs still did not point clearly to what was unfolding.

This ambiguity sits at the heart of tetanus and creates a profound ethical tension between reassurance and vigilance. Early tetanus does not arrive with a clear signature that separates it from more common and less dangerous explanations, particularly in a young puppy whose body is still learning itself. Reassurance in these contexts is not negligence. It is often responsible practice that prevents unnecessary intervention and respects the reality that bodies change and fluctuate in ways that are not always pathological.

The difficulty is that tetanus embeds itself precisely within that logic. It relies on patience, perspective, and trust in the body's capacity to regulate, using those instincts as cover while the disease progresses beneath the surface. Doubt encourages waiting, and waiting is usually rewarded when the small thing resolves, the body adapts, and the phase passes quietly. Tetanus depends on that pattern and thrives in the space where everything still looks mostly normal and escalation feels premature.

Often, the earliest warning does not come from diagnostic certainty or clinical training, but from familiarity. It comes from knowing a dog well enough to recognise when ease has been replaced by effort, even when that change cannot yet be justified or explained. Familiarity does not deliver certainty. It delivers discomfort, a persistent sense that something is not aligning with what has come before.

Responding to that discomfort requires an ethical choice that is rarely acknowledged. It requires resisting the pull toward closure and tolerating uncertainty longer than feels comfortable. It means being willing to return again and ask again, knowing that reassurance would be easier and knowing that being wrong is often more acceptable than being late.

In diseases like tetanus, where early signs are deliberately unspectacular and progression occurs beneath the surface, that kind of attentiveness does not guarantee early recognition or eliminate risk. It simply creates the possibility that something small will not be allowed to disappear because it is difficult to explain, and that possibility can matter more than certainty ever could.

Chapter 3

Being Told It Was Nothing

There is a particular kind of relief that comes from being told nothing is wrong. It is not loud or celebratory, and it does not arrive with certainty or confidence. It settles quietly, like a soft release after tension has been held just long enough to become tiring. It sounds like reassurance, but it often functions as permission. Permission to doubt your own instincts, to trust probability over unease, and to believe that the simplest explanation must be the correct one.

When the first concerns were raised, they did not arrive as panic. They arrived as questions and observations, shaped by the sense that something had shifted even if it could not yet be clearly articulated. The response to those questions was calm and professional. Nothing alarming was found. Nothing urgent was identified. Nothing obvious pointed toward serious illness. In that moment, the absence of danger felt like an answer, and that answer carried weight.

This was not negligence. It was probability.

Canine tetanus is rare. Most veterinarians will never encounter a confirmed case across their entire careers. For those who do, it may appear only once, often late in its progression and without the early warning signs that would make recognition straightforward. Veterinary medicine, like all medicine, is guided by likelihood. Clinicians are trained to consider common conditions first, not because rare diseases are ignored, but because statistically they almost never apply. Probability is not a failure of thinking. It is the foundation of safe and effective care.

Cher's veterinarian was experienced, thorough, and attentive. Her care was careful and professional, and the assessments made were reasonable based on what was visible at the time. On the first visit, Cher's eyes were examined closely. The appearance of the third eyelid was noted, but there was no sign of trauma, no obvious wound, and no indication of systemic illness. The explanation offered was irritation, with conjunctivitis suspected as the most likely cause. This was a common and sensible assumption, and eye drops were prescribed accordingly.

The drops were given as directed, but by the following day there was no improvement. That absence of response mattered, not because it signalled immediate danger, but because treatment had been initiated and observed carefully. When the expected improvement did not arrive, we returned. The second visit was not driven by alarm. It was driven by follow through. At that appointment, there was still no clear reason to move away from a common explanation. The eyes remained inflamed, the third eyelid continued to appear, and while the presentation had not escalated, it had not resolved either. No new diagnosis was made, and there was still reassurance that time and treatment would likely be sufficient.

Alongside the clinical explanations, I carried my own. The night before the first signs appeared, Cher had been bathed after doggy daycare, and I wondered whether soap or water had irritated her eyes. It felt plausible. Puppies wriggle. Water splashes. Eyes sting. There had also been a big day at the park, filled with hard play, stimulation, and fatigue. Tired puppies look different. Overstimulated puppies behave differently. A long day explains a great deal. Everything aligned in a way that felt coherent. The bath, the daycare, the park, the fatigue, the eyes. Nothing in that picture suggested something rare or dangerous.

The following day, I returned again. This was the third visit in as many days, and by then the concern was no longer about a single symptom but about consistency. The eye drops had not worked. The swelling persisted. The third eyelid continued to appear. Whatever this was, it was not resolving. At this visit, a more specific diagnosis was given. Chemosis, swelling of the conjunctival tissue, was identified as a way to account for both the appearance of her eyes and the persistence of the third eyelid. It was a clinical and reasonable conclusion, still benign, and still grounded in what was most likely.

Treatment was escalated within that diagnosis. Cher was given an injection and prescribed oral antihistamines, an appropriate next step for conjunctival inflammation that had not responded to topical treatment alone. This reflected careful, methodical medicine, the kind that follows protocol when a likely diagnosis does not immediately improve. Three visits across three consecutive days, one evolving presentation, and a diagnosis reached because symptoms persisted all pointed to a system functioning as it was designed to.

And still, there was no improvement.

The eyes remained strained. The third eyelid continued to appear in both eyes, no longer isolated or fleeting. Swelling around the eyes persisted despite escalating treatment. Her face stayed tight. Her body did not soften. Cher was not being ignored. She was being actively treated. And yet, the underlying cause remained untouched.

This is the diagnostic blind spot. When symptoms do not worsen enough to demand escalation, but do not resolve enough to reassure, they are often given time. Time is usually a friend. In tetanus, it is not.

Cher returned again, not because she was worse, but because she was unchanged. That distinction mattered. By the fourth day, I knew something had shifted, not in Cher herself, but in the situation surrounding her. We were no longer dealing with something that needed another adjustment or another period of observation. The pattern had declared itself, even though it had not yet been named.

What mattered most at that point was not the decision to refer, but the moment that made referral unavoidable. Dr Siobhan looked at Cher carefully, taking in not only the persistence of the symptoms but the coherence of the pattern they had formed across days. She then said the words that change outcomes when they are spoken with honesty and without defensiveness. She said that she *did not know what this was, that we needed help, and that a specialist was required.*

I want to be very clear about what that moment meant to me, because it is often misunderstood. What she expressed was not uncertainty in the sense of hesitation or lack of competence. It was clarity. It was the recognition that this case had moved beyond what could be responsibly managed within familiar explanations, and that continuing alone carried more risk than widening the circle of care.

It takes professional courage to recognise when experience has reached its boundary, and it takes integrity to place the animal ahead of ego, habit, or the comfort of reassurance. That decision required stepping away from what was statistically likely and acknowledging what was increasingly evident, even though it had not yet been named. I understood the significance of that choice immediately, because it altered the trajectory of everything that followed.

It was only after that decision was made that we entered the world of specialist care, and this is where Dr Emily Ireland at SASH enters Cher's story. Dr Ireland is an intensive care and neurology specialist working within a tertiary referral hospital, where complex and atypical presentations are examined through a different lens. Her involvement did not represent a sudden solution or dramatic escalation, but the necessary extension of care once the limits of general probability had been reached.

That singular decision to look beyond individual experience and seek additional expertise is the moment my dog was saved. Not because the answer was suddenly known or immediately visible, but because time was no longer being spent waiting for reassurance to become resolution. In conditions like tetanus, time does not behave generously, and the disease does not announce itself kindly. What mattered was that care moved forward before certainty arrived, guided by responsibility rather than comfort.

In moments like this, the most powerful decision in medicine is not the ability to name the answer quickly or to persist alone in the absence of clarity. It is the discernment to recognise when a case has moved beyond the safe limits of individual experience, and the willingness to ask for help while that help can still change the outcome. That choice is where reassurance gives way to leadership, and where medicine, at its best, becomes a collaborative act grounded in humility, judgement, and care.

Chapter 4

The Question That Would Not Leave

There is a moment that comes after reassurance has been given, after explanations have been offered, and after logic has done everything, it is supposed to do. It is the moment when the words sound reasonable, the plan makes sense, and the professionals involved appear calm and competent, and yet something still does not sit properly. That moment does not arrive with urgency or clarity. It does not announce itself as certainty. It arrives quietly, as a persistent discomfort that refuses to resolve simply because it has been addressed.

Instinct is often misunderstood as emotion, anxiety, or overreaction, particularly when it appears in the absence of evidence. But instinct is not panic. It is pattern recognition without language. It is the nervous system noticing deviation before the mind has gathered enough information to explain it. It operates beneath conscious reasoning, drawing on familiarity, repetition, and lived experience rather than data points or diagnostic labels.

By the fourth day, I did not have proof. I did not have a diagnosis, test results, or a clear name for what was happening.

What I did have was something far more specific than suspicion. I had baseline knowledge. That knowledge did not come from training or expertise. It came from proximity.

People who live closely with animals develop this understanding slowly and without ceremony. A dog has a rhythm, a way of moving through the world that becomes deeply familiar over time. There is a normal expression, a normal degree of softness, a predictable pattern of energy, recovery, and rest. You learn how your dog looks when they are relaxed, how they settle after play, how their eyes soften when they are tired, and how quickly they return to themselves after stimulation. This kind of knowing is not theoretical. It is embodied.

Cher was not returning to baseline. She was not softening, settling, or resetting after rest or treatment. Every reasonable explanation had been applied, and every logical treatment had been trialled. And still her body held its tension. Her eyes remained strained, her face stayed tight, the third eyelid continued to appear in both eyes, and the swelling did not recede. This was not escalation, but it was persistence, and persistence without resolution is where instinct begins to speak.

Instinct does not live in hysteria. It lives in contrast. It arises when today does not match yesterday, when this walk does not resemble the last one, and when rest no longer looks like rest. Dog owners who truly know their animals are not searching for drama or rare diagnoses, and they are not attempting to outthink professionals. They are noticing difference. They are comparing patterns across days rather than moments, and when those comparisons no longer align, something registers even if it cannot yet be explained.

Trusting instinct does not mean rejecting expertise. It means recognising when expertise has reached the edge of probability, when the most likely explanations have been exhausted and the picture still does not fit. I did not know it was tetanus, and I want to be clear about that. What I knew was simpler and harder to dismiss. This was not normal. This was not resolving. This was not how my dog behaved.

That clarity mattered. Good advocacy is not about volume or insistence. It is about precision. It is the ability to articulate what has changed, what is missing, and what is no longer present. It is about being able to say that something is different even when you cannot yet say why. The most effective advocates are calm, consistent, and observant. They return not because things are dramatically worse, but because they are unchanged. They understand their animal well enough to recognise when a presentation sits outside that animal's normal range.

This is not nuisance behaviour. It is responsible care.

When Dr Siobhan said that she did not know what this was, I felt relief rather than fear. Her words aligned with what my instincts had already been telling me. Something else was at play. Trusting instinct in that moment meant agreeing to widen the lens. It meant saying yes to referral, yes to escalation, and yes to specialist care even without a diagnosis in hand.

This is the point at which many people hesitate. Without proof, it can feel uncomfortable to push forward. Without certainty, insisting on more can feel unreasonable, particularly when reassurance has already been offered by someone trained, experienced, and calm. But instinct does not demand proof. It demands honesty. It asks a single question, *Is this right?*

In Cher's case, the answer was no.

Trusting instinct did not mean accusing anyone of being wrong or dismissing medical advice. It meant acknowledging that the current frame was no longer sufficient. Instinct is not opposition to medicine. It is often the mechanism that brings medicine to the right place. Rare conditions do not announce themselves clearly, and they do not fit neatly into early diagnostic categories. They rely on someone noticing that the pattern is off even when each individual piece still appears plausible.

This is why instinct matters most when proof is absent. By the time proof arrives, instinct is no longer required because the body has already declared itself. In tetanus, waiting for proof often means waiting too long.

What helped to save Cher was not certainty. It was movement. It was advocacy grounded in familiarity rather than fear. It was the refusal to stop simply because reassurance had been given when the body in front of us had not yet returned to itself.

Sometimes trusting instinct is not about knowing what is wrong. It is about knowing that stopping would mean accepting an explanation that no longer fits, and choosing instead to remain attentive until the picture finally makes sense.

.

PART II:

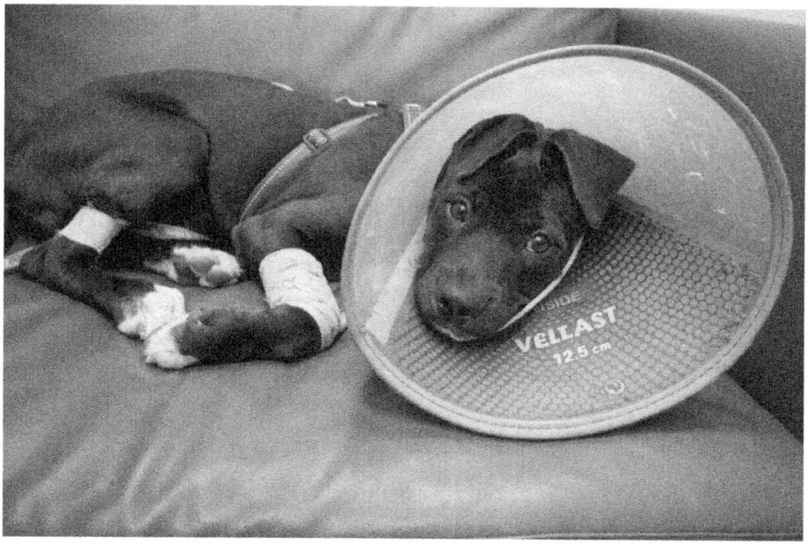

THE DIAGNOSIS NO ONE EXPECTS

Up until this point, everything in Cher's story still lived comfortably within the realm of the ordinary. The explanations offered were familiar and reassuring, grounded in conditions that veterinarians and dog owners encounter every day. Irritation was plausible. Inflammation made sense. Allergy was reasonable. Fatigue fit easily into the context of a young, active puppy still finding her limits. Even developmental variation provided a framework that felt safe and explanatory. Each possibility stood on its own with credibility, and together they formed a picture that did not challenge expectation.

Nothing about what had unfolded so far sounded rare. Nothing carried the weight of catastrophe or the gravity of a diagnosis that changes the temperature of a room. There were no dramatic collapses, no obvious wounds, and no sudden crises that demanded immediate reclassification of what was happening. The story, as it stood, was one most people would recognise and find comfort in. That familiarity was precisely what made the next stage so dangerous.

Tetanus does not announce itself early. It does not arrive with spectacle or clarity, and it does not offer the kinds of signs people are taught to fear. Instead, it hides behind what looks reasonable and expected, borrowing the language of common conditions and ordinary variation. By the time it is named, it is often already advanced. By the time it is suspected, it has usually had time to interfere deeply with the nervous system. By the time the word is spoken aloud, many dogs do not survive.

Most veterinarians will never encounter a confirmed case of canine tetanus across their entire careers. Most dog owners will never hear the diagnosis spoken in relation to their own animal. It does not sit on the list of conditions people anticipate, plan for, or actively watch for. That rarity is often treated as reassurance, but in reality it is deceptive. Rare does not mean impossible. It means unexpected, and unexpected diagnoses are often the ones most likely to slip through the cracks created by probability, reassurance, and reasonable explanations.

Everything that happened before this point matters because it is what allowed the unexpected to be seen at all. The early signs that did not resolve, the persistence across days rather than moments, the repeated visits that were driven by consistency rather than panic, and the refusal to accept that unchanged meant improving all contributed to what followed. So did the willingness to widen the circle of care before certainty arrived. Without those steps, what came next would not have been recognised in time.

This is the point at which the story shifts. The uncertainty that has been carefully held gives way to clarity that arrives suddenly and without comfort. Reassurance is replaced by reckoning, and instinct finally meets diagnosis. The word that follows is one most people associate with rusted metal, deep wounds, and human medicine rather than veterinary neurology. Almost no one expects it to apply to a puppy. Almost no one expects it to be survivable. Almost no one expects to hear it spoken during a specialist consultation about a young dog who, until recently, still looked mostly normal.

And yet, this is where Cher's story goes next.

Chapter 5

When the Word Tetanus Appears

From my vet, we went straight to SASH. Dr Siobhan had already sent a detailed referral letter ahead, including her consult notes and observations from the previous days. There was no delay and no gap in care. The handover had begun before I even turned the key in the ignition, and that continuity mattered more than I understood at the time.

The drive took only thirty minutes, but it felt far longer. In that short stretch of road, my mind raced ahead of reality, filling the absence of information with imagined catastrophes. I convinced myself that she was dying. I imagined brain tumours, unseen head injuries at doggy daycare, and irreversible damage that no one had detected in time. I tried to prepare myself for devastation, rehearsing grief before it arrived in the hope that it might hurt less when it did.

What I did not know then was that nothing I imagined would come close to the reality of what was about to unfold.

When I arrived at SASH, the first thing that struck me was not fear. It was surprise. The waiting room did not resemble the sterile, rushed spaces I associated with medical crisis. It was calm, considered, and quietly extraordinary. The design, the flow, the reception staff, and the attention to detail all communicated competence and care without urgency or drama. Everything about the space suggested that difficult things happened here regularly, and that they were handled with intention. That steadiness mattered more than I realised at the time.

I was shown into a small, open, private holding cubicle with Cher. It was a quiet space with just enough separation from the rest of the clinic to allow me to breathe. There was no pressure to perform calmness, but also no chaos. I held onto that stillness tightly.

Then the triage nurse came out. She took one look at Cher. It was not a prolonged assessment or a careful examination, but a glance informed by experience. Calmly and without hesitation, she said that Cher was a tetanus dog. For a moment, the words did not register. My mind stalled as it tried to reconcile that sentence with everything I thought I knew.

She explained that she needed to take Cher out the back to confirm with a veterinarian. There was no alarm in her voice and no urgency in her movements. Cher was lifted gently and carried away, and suddenly the room felt very empty. When she returned, the confirmation was clear. Cher had tetanus.

That was how the word appeared.

It landed all at once and fractured time. Part of me remained standing in the room, listening and nodding, trying to stay upright and present. Another part of me had already moved far ahead, spiralling into everything that word carried with it. Tetanus was heavy with implication. It was a word most people associate with rusted metal, deep wounds, and human medicine. It did not belong in a puppy. It did not belong in this story.

As Cher was taken away again, I was left in the waiting room with nothing but my phone, my thoughts, and a name for the thing that had been stalking us quietly for days. This was where modern medicine collided with modern information. ChatGPT became both companion and tormentor. Google became both lifeline and enemy. Google Scholar offered evidence and fear in equal measure. I searched obsessively, trying to orient myself inside a reality I had not expected to enter.

I read about case fatality rates, delayed diagnosis, neurological progression, muscle rigidity, and respiratory failure. Every answer opened three more questions. Every hopeful sentence carried a qualifier that tightened my chest. Survival was possible, but rare. Recovery could happen, but not without risk. Outcomes depended on timing, severity, access to antitoxin, and intensive care. I was learning in real time that tetanus is not just a disease. It is a waiting game, and waiting is brutal.

Around me, the room carried its own quiet stories. Conversations were low and careful. Eyes were red from crying. People held carriers that were suddenly too still. Names were called that did not return. Veterinary waiting rooms hold a particular kind of grief. It is intimate and unfiltered, and there is no expectation that everything will be fine.

When I was finally taken through to speak with the specialist, I met Dr Emily Ireland. We sat together in that room for a long time, close to half an hour, although time behaved strangely by then and the exact shape of the conversation has since blurred. What I remember is not a list of questions or answers, but the way the space felt once she began to speak.

Every question I had already asked the internet was asked again, out loud, even if I no longer remember the words themselves. Dr Emily answered each one calmly and directly, without minimising the seriousness of the diagnosis and without inflating fear. She was clear that tetanus is difficult to treat, not because there is no protocol, but because risk sits on top of risk, and complications can emerge even when everything is done correctly. She did not soften that truth or offer false comfort.

At the same time, she was quietly confident in her own ability to treat Cher. There was no bravado in that confidence, and no promise of outcome. What she offered instead was something far more grounded. She told me that she could not guarantee success, but that she would do everything within her veterinary power to save my dog. That was the only promise she made, and it was the one that mattered.

In that moment, honesty was more reassuring than certainty could ever have been. I did not need to be told that everything would be fine. I needed to know that Cher was in the hands of someone who understood the disease, respected its unpredictability, and was willing to meet it fully.

Not long after that conversation, another realisation arrived with uncomfortable clarity. Years earlier, I had made the decision to invest in top tier pet insurance, not because I expected catastrophe, but because I never wanted cost to be the reason I hesitated. Sitting there in that room, that decision mattered. There was no internal debate about whether we could proceed, no calculation about whether treatment was worth it, and no pause to weigh money against time. Care could move when it needed to move.

My role became simple. I needed to love my girl, be present, trust the people treating her, and keep my focus on her recovery rather than on invoices. That clarity matters more than people realise. When a pet is critically ill, decision fatigue can cost precious time, and hesitation compounds fear. Resources become another burden to carry. I did not have to fight that battle, and my energy could stay where it belonged, with Cher.

What complicated matters further was the reality that tetanus antitoxin is not something most small animal hospitals keep on hand, particularly in major cities where the disease is rarely seen. Demand is low and supply is limited. This was the week before Christmas. Suppliers were closing, it was after hours, and time was not on our side. Tetanus does not wait, and every hour matters.

And yet, the system held.

The antitoxin was sourced, the treatment plan moved forward, and care continued without delay. In that moment, I understood something with absolute clarity. Cher was not saved by luck alone. She was not saved by one person, one drug, or one decision. She was saved because the chain of care did not break.

A concern was noticed early and voiced. A veterinarian recognised the limits of certainty and escalated. A specialist met the disease with honesty and skill. A system responded quickly. Treatment was accessed without hesitation. Each link held, and if any one of those moments had failed, the outcome would likely have been different.

This is not a story about heroics. It is a story about continuity, humility, and systems that work when the people inside them are willing to act. That is what saved her.

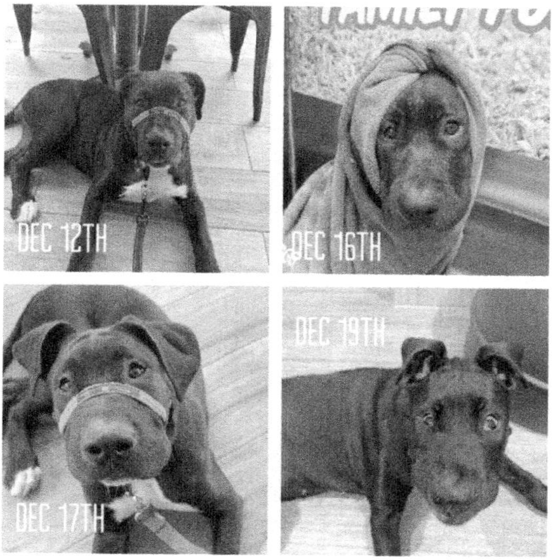

The changes in Cher within a week.
Admitted to ICU 19th December 2025

Chapter 6

How Tetanus Hides in Plain Sight

Tetanus is not a disease of dramatic entry. In dogs, it does not arrive with spectacle or a clear moment of failure. There is no sudden collapse, no obvious wound that demands attention, and no single event that clearly marks the beginning of illness. Instead, tetanus enters quietly, through a series of small and often forgettable encounters that only gain meaning in hindsight. This subtlety is not incidental. It is fundamental to the biology of the disease.

Tetanus is caused by Clostridium tetani, a spore-forming, anaerobic bacterium that exists widely in the natural environment. The spores are exceptionally resilient and can persist in soil for years, surviving heat, desiccation, and many common disinfectants. Veterinary and medical literature has long established that C. tetani is not rare in nature. What is rare is the precise convergence of conditions required for it to cause disease. This distinction matters, because most dogs encounter tetanus spores repeatedly throughout their lives without consequence. Exposure alone is not the problem. Disease occurs only when exposure is paired with opportunity.

The true danger lies not in the bacterium itself, but in the toxin it produces. When Clostridium tetani enters a wound environment that supports its growth, it can begin producing tetanospasmin, one of the most potent neurotoxins known. Unlike many infectious diseases, tetanus does not rely on bacterial spread throughout the body. The organism can remain localised at the site of entry while the toxin travels silently along peripheral nerves toward the spinal cord and brainstem. This process, known as retrograde axonal transport, is slow and deliberate. It does not trigger the immune system in a way that produces fever, inflammation, or obvious systemic illness. Blood tests are often unremarkable, and imaging frequently reveals nothing of concern. The disease progresses beneath the threshold of routine detection.

Once the toxin reaches the central nervous system, it interferes with inhibitory neurotransmitters, particularly glycine and gamma-aminobutyric acid. These neurotransmitters are responsible for telling muscles when to relax. When their function is blocked, muscles receive only one message. They are instructed to contract, but never to release. This mechanism explains why tetanus presents as rigidity rather than weakness, stiffness rather than paralysis, and sustained tension rather than collapse in its early stages. It also explains why the disease is so often misinterpreted. The dog is not floppy or unresponsive. Instead, the body appears to be working too hard, locked into effort.

For tetanus to develop, several conditions usually have to align. Veterinary case series and reviews consistently demonstrate that when one of these elements is missing, disease does not occur. The first requirement is a break in the skin, although it rarely looks like the kind of injury people expect. In fact, the literature repeatedly notes that the inciting wound is often minor or never identified at all. Small punctures, healing scratches, paw pad abrasions, oral lesions, and facial scrapes are common points of entry. In puppies, these injuries are particularly easy to overlook. Puppies fall, scrape, chew, and collide with their environment as part of normal development. Their skin heals quickly, pain responses are brief, and visible signs often disappear almost as fast as they appear. In many documented cases of canine tetanus, no wound is ever found.

The second condition is exposure to an environment where tetanus spores are present in sufficient quantity. These spores are most abundant in soil rich in organic matter, particularly where animal waste is present. Agricultural and veterinary literature has long associated tetanus with horse environments, including paddocks, stables, and agistment areas, but similar risk profiles exist elsewhere. Muddy creeks, dams, stagnant water, and wet sediment create low-oxygen microenvironments that allow spores to persist. Dogs do not need direct contact with livestock. Running, digging, swimming, or walking through contaminated ground is enough to facilitate exposure. Importantly, these environments are not unusual or extreme. They are ordinary places where dogs are meant to be.

Exposure alone, however, is still not enough. The most critical factor is the creation of a low-oxygen wound environment. Clostridium tetani cannot thrive in the presence of oxygen. Small wounds that close quickly can trap bacteria beneath the skin, creating ideal conditions for toxin production. By the time the surface appears healed, oxygen tension may have dropped below the threshold that suppresses bacterial activity. This paradox is well documented in both veterinary and human medicine. Clean, fast-healing wounds may pose greater risk than open injuries that allow oxygen exposure and drainage. This alone explains why tetanus often appears to come from nowhere.

Time is the next essential ingredient. Tetanus does not progress in a way that forces early recognition. The toxin moves slowly along nerves, resulting in an incubation period that can range from several days to several weeks. During this time, there may be no visible signs of infection, no systemic illness, and no abnormalities on routine testing. When clinical signs finally emerge, they do so gradually. Subtle stiffness, facial tension, changes in posture, difficulty relaxing, and altered gait are easy to attribute to musculoskeletal strain, behavioural change, or developmental phases, particularly in young dogs. By the time tetanus is suspected, the toxin may already be well established within the nervous system.

The final factor is the absence of protective immunity. Dogs are not routinely vaccinated against tetanus. This is not an oversight. Dogs are generally more resistant to tetanus than humans, and the disease occurs infrequently enough that routine vaccination has not been considered necessary. Resistance, however, does not equal immunity. When sufficient toxin is produced and reaches the central nervous system, that resistance can be overcome. Veterinary case reviews consistently show that when tetanus occurs in dogs, it is often severe, prolonged, and requires intensive supportive care. Recovery, when it occurs, can take weeks to months.

Taken together, these factors explain why tetanus is so often missed. It is not missed because veterinarians are careless or inattentive. It is missed because the disease is structured to evade early recognition. From a clinical perspective, tetanus presents in a way that conflicts with expectation. Most neurological emergencies arrive loudly, with collapse, seizures, loss of consciousness, or dramatic behavioural change. Tetanus does none of these things at first. Early signs are subtle, localised, and easy to explain away. Facial tension is treated as ocular irritation. Stiffness is attributed to muscle strain. Changes in gait are labelled orthopaedic or developmental. In puppies, normal growth further masks abnormal progression.

Rarity compounds the problem. Most veterinarians will never encounter a confirmed case of canine tetanus in their careers. Rare diagnoses are not absent, but they are easily outranked by more common explanations. The absence of a visible wound further reduces suspicion, and the lack of early diagnostic clarity reinforces reassurance. Blood work is often normal. Imaging is unrevealing. The toxin does not circulate in a way that can be easily measured. Diagnosis is clinical, based on pattern recognition, progression over time, and exclusion of other causes.

This places extraordinary importance on two things: time and familiarity. Time reveals progression, and familiarity reveals deviation from baseline. Owners who know their dog's normal posture, expression, movement, and behaviour are often the first to notice when something does not resolve. Diagnosis is rarely missed because someone failed to look. It is missed because what they saw still looked reasonable, until it no longer did.

By the time tetanus is suspected, the disease has often progressed beyond its earliest stage. This is why intensive care is so frequently required, and why outcomes depend so heavily on how quickly the diagnosis is finally made. Escalation matters because tetanus is not found early by certainty. It is found early by recognising when uncertainty no longer fits.

Understanding how tetanus occurs is not about fear or restriction. Dogs should run, dig, swim, and explore. These activities are essential to their physical and psychological health. Awareness is not about avoidance. It is about recognising that when subtle neurological signs appear days or weeks later, the story often began long before anyone thought to look. Tetanus does not announce itself. It waits.

How Cher contracted tetanus will likely never be known. There was no obvious wound, no single event that could be pointed to as the beginning, and no clear explanation that neatly accounts for what followed. This is not unusual. In many cases of canine tetanus, the point of entry is never identified, and searching for it rarely changes what matters. By the time the disease is recognised, the conditions that allowed it to take hold are already in the past. What determines outcome is not where tetanus began, but how quickly it was recognised and responded to once it did.

Chapter 7

ICU

Intensive Care Units (ICU) are not just for people. In veterinary medicine, an ICU exists for the same reason it does in human hospitals. It exists to support bodies that cannot support themselves, to monitor systems that can no longer be left unattended, and to intervene quickly when small changes carry disproportionate consequence. For dogs, ICU is not a room or a ward in the way most people imagine. It is a level of care defined by vigilance, precision, and sustained attention.

ICU care means continuous monitoring rather than periodic checks, frequent reassessment rather than assumptions of stability, and the capacity to respond immediately when a parameter shifts, even subtly. Breathing, hydration, nutrition, temperature regulation, muscle tone, pain, and comfort are all actively managed rather than passively observed. Nothing is left to chance, and nothing is assumed to be self-correcting.

Dogs are admitted to ICU when their condition is unstable, unpredictable, or at risk of rapid deterioration. Neurological disease, severe infection, respiratory compromise, and systemic illness are among the most common reasons. These are conditions where the margin for error is narrow and where delay carries consequence.

Tetanus sits squarely within this category.

Once tetanus is diagnosed, the body becomes a site of sustained physiological strain. Muscles that cannot relax consume energy relentlessly. The constant state of contraction generates heat, fatigue, and pain. Breathing can become compromised as chest wall muscles stiffen. Swallowing may become unsafe as jaw and throat muscles lose coordination. External stimulation, even gentle handling, can trigger painful spasms that further exhaust the body. The nervous system remains trapped in activation, unable to downshift.

ICU care exists to reduce these risks while the body undertakes the slow work of recovery. There is no medication that instantly reverses tetanus once the toxin has bound to nerve endings. Recovery depends on time, nerve regeneration, and careful support while the toxin's effects gradually diminish. ICU does not cure tetanus. It creates the conditions in which survival becomes possible.

For pet owners, ICU is overwhelming in ways that are difficult to anticipate. It represents the sudden loss of physical access to your animal. The shock of handover happens quickly, often before the reality has fully settled. One moment you are holding your dog, reading her signals and adjusting her comfort, and the next you are stepping back while someone else takes over completely.

You go from being the primary carer to being a visitor, and sometimes not even that. Decisions are made rapidly. Information arrives in dense, technical language. Updates are measured and careful, designed to inform without alarming. There are rules around visiting, infection control, and stimulation, all designed to protect the patient rather than the emotional needs of the person who loves them.

ICU also carries symbolic weight. The word itself signals seriousness. It marks a threshold crossed, a moment when outpatient care and observation are no longer sufficient. It forces a confrontation with uncertainty and with the limits of control. For many owners, ICU is the first time they are asked to fully accept that loving an animal does not guarantee outcome.

And yet, ICU is also where time is bought.

It is where bodies are given the space to heal without being overwhelmed by their own limitations. It is where vigilance replaces guessing, and where intervention is available the moment it is needed rather than after something has already gone wrong. ICU is not the end of the story. It is the place where the work becomes deliberate, where waiting becomes structured, and where hope exists in fragile but meaningful form.

This is where Cher went next.

ICU begins with separation. There is no gentle transition into it. There is no easing in. One moment your dog is with you, and the next she is carried through a door marked *Staff Only*. You do not walk out with her. You walk out without her, and the absence is immediate and physical.

In veterinary medicine, ICU is the point reached when a body can no longer be trusted to regulate itself safely. For Cher, that threshold was crossed quickly once tetanus was confirmed. Her muscles were no longer able to rest. The toxin had locked them into contraction, draining energy continuously. Stimulation triggered spasms. Swallowing could not be assumed to be safe. Breathing required close observation.

What her body needed most was time, protection from additional stress, and care that could adapt minute by minute.

The first day in ICU is not about improvement. It is about containment and stability. The goal is to prevent deterioration while the body absorbs the reality of what is happening.

Cher was sedated to reduce muscle rigidity and prevent painful spasms. Sedation in tetanus is not about rendering a dog unconscious. It is about lowering the nervous system's responsiveness so that the body is not constantly fighting itself. The balance is delicate. Too little sedation allows spasms to break through, increasing pain and exhaustion. Too much sedation suppresses breathing, reflexes, and protective responses. Every adjustment is made cautiously and reviewed continuously.

She was placed in a low stimulus environment designed to minimise triggers. Lighting was dim. Noise was controlled. Handling was kept to what was strictly necessary. In tetanus, calm is not comfort. Calm is treatment. Even well-intentioned touch can provoke muscle contraction, so restraint becomes part of care.

I learned very quickly that ICU medicine is not dramatic. It is meticulous. It is a series of small decisions made carefully and revisited often.

That first night stretched endlessly. Updates came in measured language. Stable. No deterioration. Holding. These words became anchors, not because they promised recovery, but because they meant nothing had been lost.

The second day in ICU brings a different reality. The adrenaline of diagnosis fades, replaced by the understanding that recovery will not be quick. Tetanus does not resolve in days. It resolves in weeks, sometimes months. The timeline is long, and the work is incremental.

Cher remained under constant observation. Her breathing pattern was assessed repeatedly. Muscle tone was evaluated across different parts of her body. Swallow reflexes were checked carefully before any attempt at feeding. Hydration was maintained through intravenous fluids to reduce strain and prevent dehydration in a body already working too hard.

There were no breakthroughs. There were no setbacks. In ICU, that absence of change is often the best possible outcome.

For owners, this stage is particularly difficult. There is nothing to react to and nothing to celebrate. There is no crisis to respond to and no clear milestone to mark. You exist in a suspended state where waiting becomes the primary task.

By the third day and beyond, the smallest changes begin to matter. A muscle that softens slightly when repositioned. A spasm that resolves more quickly than it did the day before. A posture that looks marginally less rigid. These are changes most people would never notice. In ICU, they are observed, documented, discussed, and used to guide subtle adjustments in care.

Cher's sedation was modified in response to these signs. ICU care is never static. Medications are titrated continuously. Comfort is reassessed. Risk is recalculated. The aim is always to support without pushing, to protect without suppressing recovery.

I learned that ICU is often less about intervention than it is about restraint. Knowing when not to advance. Knowing when not to reduce support too quickly. Knowing when to let the body lead rather than forcing progress.

Visits, when they were allowed, were some of the hardest moments of the entire experience.

Cher was not connected to blinking monitors or surrounded by the constant alarms people often associate with intensive care. Instead, her body told the story plainly. Thin tubes ran into her nose. Every available limb was wrapped and rewrapped, bearing the marks of needles, intravenous lines, and repeated access points. Her body had become a map of intervention, each bandage evidence of how much support she required simply to hold herself together.

When I was brought into the patient visiting room, Cher was walked in to meet me. She moved stiffly and awkwardly, her body rigid in a way that was foreign to a young puppy. She was confused and clearly unwell, disoriented by medication, by unfamiliar surroundings, and by the effort required simply to exist inside a body that would not soften.

She wanted closeness and reassurance, but her muscles could not tolerate touch for long. She wanted movement, but movement triggered discomfort. She wanted to settle, but her body resisted release. What she wanted most was simple and heartbreaking in its ordinariness. She wanted to lie down and rest.

Watching her navigate those competing needs was devastating. She leaned into me, then pulled away. She sought comfort, then stiffened when contact became too much. Her desire for reassurance collided constantly with the physical limitations imposed by tetanus. Even love became complicated. Even touch carried consequence.

The visits themselves were emotionally brutal in another way as well. Each one came with the knowledge that it would end. That soon I would have to stand up, hand her back, and walk out without her again. The drive home after each visit was a quiet endurance exercise, filled with hope and fear in equal measure. I replayed every small observation, searching for signs of improvement while trying not to catastrophise the absence of obvious change.

Because Cher was still a young puppy and newly part of our family, another worry sat alongside the medical fear. I worried about bonding. I worried about what was being lost during this critical time when connection is usually built through shared routines, play, and constant physical presence. Instead, her earliest weeks with us were marked by separation, illness, and restraint. That loss felt profound and unfair, even as I knew there was no alternative.

It was hard on me. It was hard on Elton, who could not understand where she had gone or why the house felt wrong without her. But most of all, it was hard on Cher. She was sick, frightened, rigid, and confused, navigating pain and disorientation at an age when the world should still feel safe and predictable.

ICU protected her body, but it could not protect her from the emotional cost of being unwell and separated from everything familiar.

And still, it was the right place for her to be.

As the days continued, progress did not move in straight lines. Some signs improved while others plateaued. The care team remained cautious. Tetanus is unpredictable, and overconfidence carries risk.

Feeding remained a particular concern, as swallowing difficulties are common due to rigidity in the jaw and throat. Nutrition had to be managed carefully to avoid aspiration while ensuring her body had the resources it needed to heal. Every system was being supported so that no single failure would overwhelm the rest.

Gradually and almost imperceptibly, Cher began to change. Muscle tone softened. Periods of alertness increased. Her body began to rest rather than brace. These changes were fragile and required protection. Sedation was reduced slowly. Monitoring continued without pause. Setbacks were anticipated rather than feared and understood as part of the process rather than evidence of failure.

By this stage, ICU no longer felt like crisis. It felt like endurance. For owners, this brings a different kind of exhaustion. Hope returns, but it is careful and contained. You learn not to ask how long it will take. You learn to accept that healing happens on the body's timetable, not yours.

ICU taught me something fundamental.
Cher was not fighting tetanus. Her body was.

The role of ICU was to make sure she had the space, safety, and support to do that work without being overwhelmed.

Chapter 8

What Treatment Really Looks Like

When people hear the word treatment, they often imagine something decisive. They picture a drug that fixes the problem, a procedure that reverses the damage, or a clear turning point where fear finally gives way to relief. This expectation comes from how most illnesses behave. Infection is treated, inflammation settles, healing follows. Tetanus does not follow that pattern. There is no single medication that cures it and no intervention that immediately undoes what the toxin has already done. Treatment is not a switch that gets flipped. It is a process that unfolds slowly, often invisibly, over time, and it demands a kind of patience that feels unnatural when fear is still present.

The reason tetanus defies expectations lies in how the disease works. By the time tetanus is diagnosed, the bacteria that caused it may already be inactive or confined to a tiny, often undetectable site. The illness is no longer driven by infection in the traditional sense. It is driven by a toxin that has already travelled along nerves and interfered with the body's ability to regulate muscle movement. This is why tetanus behaves so differently from most infections. The damage is neurological, not bacterial, and neurological systems do not heal quickly.

Antibiotics are still used, but their purpose is preventative rather than curative. They are given to eliminate any remaining *Clostridium tetani* bacteria and to stop further toxin production. In some cases, a wound can be identified and treated directly. In many cases, no wound is ever found. This is not unusual. The bacteria can enter through microscopic breaks in the skin that heal before anyone notices them. Antibiotics can stop new harm from occurring, but they cannot reverse harm that has already occurred. Once the toxin has entered the nervous system, antibiotics no longer change the course of the disease.

Antitoxin works on a similar principle. It can neutralise toxin that is still circulating in the body, but it cannot detach toxin that has already bound to nerve endings. This binding is what causes the characteristic muscle rigidity and spasms of tetanus. Once the toxin is attached, the body must wait for nerve terminals to regenerate and re-establish normal inhibitory signalling. This biological process takes time. There is no medication that can accelerate it. This is why early recognition matters so profoundly, and why even a short delay can change outcomes.

Even when antibiotics and antitoxin are administered promptly, they represent only a small part of treatment because they address only what can still be stopped. They do not address what is already happening. That work falls to supportive care.

Supportive care is the cornerstone of tetanus treatment because the body must be supported while the nervous system heals itself. The toxin blocks inhibitory neurotransmitters that normally tell muscles when to relax. Without those signals, muscles remain locked in a state of contraction. This constant contraction is not only painful, it is metabolically exhausting. Muscles consume oxygen continuously when they cannot relax, which is why oxygen levels must be monitored closely. Increased oxygen demand combined with restricted chest movement can lead to respiratory compromise if not managed carefully.

Sedation is used because it dampens excessive nerve firing and reduces muscle activity. It does not cure the disease, but it protects the body from the consequences of uncontrolled contraction. Sedation must be carefully titrated because too little allows spasms to persist, while too much can suppress breathing. This balance changes as the disease evolves, which is why sedation plans are reviewed constantly rather than set once.

Spasms are common because the nervous system becomes hypersensitive when inhibitory pathways are disrupted. Normal stimuli that would usually be filtered out become overwhelming. Light, sound, touch, and sudden movement can all trigger exaggerated muscle responses. This is why environmental control is not simply a comfort measure but a medical necessity. Reducing stimulation lowers the likelihood of spasms and decreases metabolic strain on the body. Calm becomes treatment because calm reduces neurological demand.

Breathing requires continuous attention because the muscles involved in respiration are not exempt from tetanus. When chest wall muscles remain rigid, breathing becomes shallow and inefficient. Over time, respiratory muscles can fatigue under the strain of constant contraction. Monitoring oxygen levels allows clinicians to intervene before fatigue becomes failure. In severe cases, mechanical support is used not because the lungs are diseased, but because the muscles controlling them are overwhelmed.

Swallowing is affected for the same neurological reason. The muscles of the jaw, throat, and upper oesophagus rely on precise coordination between contraction and relaxation. When inhibitory signals are disrupted, that coordination breaks down. Swallowing becomes unsafe, and the risk of aspiration rises sharply. This is why feeding is delayed or modified and why hydration is often provided intravenously. These decisions are protective, not regressive, and they are revisited repeatedly as function slowly returns.

Temperature dysregulation occurs because constant muscle contraction generates heat, sometimes leading to fever without infection. At the same time, prolonged immobility and sedation can impair the body's ability to maintain warmth. Active temperature management is required because the body's usual regulatory mechanisms are compromised.

Pain in tetanus is multifaceted. It arises from sustained muscle contraction, repeated spasms, and the strain of immobility. Pain management is complex because pain itself can increase muscle tension and trigger spasms, creating a feedback loop. Effective pain control reduces this loop but must be balanced carefully to avoid excessive sedation.

Recovery from tetanus is slow because nerve healing is slow. The toxin does not damage nerves in a way that can be repaired overnight. Inhibitory pathways must regenerate, and synaptic function must be restored. This process varies between individuals. It depends on how much toxin bound to the nervous system, which nerves were affected, how early treatment began, and how the individual body responds. This is why there is no single timeline for recovery and why every dog's course looks different.

Progress is rarely linear because nerve recovery does not occur uniformly. Some pathways recover before others. One muscle group may relax while another remains rigid. A reflex may return and then falter as the system recalibrates. These fluctuations are expected. They do not signal failure. They signal adaptation.

Setbacks are common because prolonged illness creates vulnerability. Fatigue accumulates. Secondary infections can occur. Aspiration remains a risk even as swallowing improves. Immobility can lead to pressure injuries or gastrointestinal disturbances. These setbacks are not evidence that treatment is ineffective. They are recognised risks of a long recovery and are the reason tetanus is managed in intensive care settings whenever possible.

Owners almost always ask the same question: when will I see improvement? They ask it because uncertainty is exhausting, and because human experience tells us that treatment should have a visible endpoint. The honest answer remains the same. Improvement is slow because healing is slow. The first goal is survival. The second is stability. Improvement comes later, often quietly and incrementally.

Treatment is about holding the body steady long enough for the nervous system to recover. It is about preventing avoidable harm while allowing unavoidable processes to unfold. There is no dramatic turning point, no single marker of success. Progress reveals itself only when looked back upon.

This is what treatment really looks like. Not a cure. Not a rescue. Not a dramatic turnaround.

It is a commitment.

A commitment to consistency, vigilance, and patience. Cher did not recover because one medication worked. She recovered because every element of her care worked together, day after day, while her body did the slow work it needed to do. That is what tetanus demands. And that is what treatment truly is.

PART III:

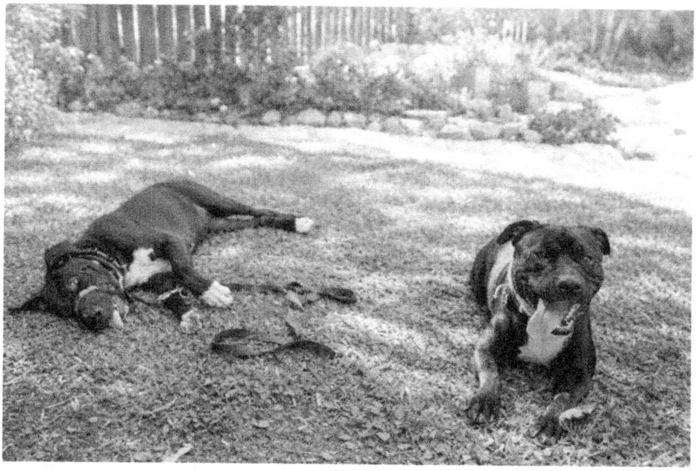

The Long Middle

There is a moment in serious illness when the language changes, and it often arrives quietly enough that people barely notice it at first.

The urgency that once filled every interaction begins to recede. The alarms that demanded immediate attention grow less frequent. Conversations no longer revolve around crisis protocols or emergency thresholds. Words like *critical* and *unstable* begin to disappear from the daily updates. In their place come words that sound gentler, steadier, almost comforting. Stabilised. Managed. Improving. These words are not offered lightly. They are spoken with care, with professionalism, and often with genuine relief. They signal that the body is no longer tipping toward catastrophe.

For many people, this shift in language is interpreted as the beginning of relief.

It feels like permission to exhale. Like confirmation that the worst has passed. Like the moment when fear should begin to loosen its grip and hope should finally have room to grow.

In tetanus, this moment does not function the way people expect it to.

The point at which a patient becomes stabilised is not the point at which the danger is over. It is the point at which the work changes shape. The emergency phase recedes, but it does not resolve into recovery. Instead, it opens into a long and demanding stretch of time that sits between survival and healing, a phase that has no neat clinical label but defines the lived experience of the illness more than any other.

This is the long middle.

The long middle is not the beginning, when urgency clarifies priorities and decisive action feels possible. It is not the end, when progress becomes visible and recovery can be measured in milestones. It is the prolonged in between, where nothing is actively worsening, yet very little appears to be getting better. Days begin to resemble one another. Care routines repeat. The absence of deterioration becomes the primary marker of success, even as visible improvement remains elusive.

Stabilised does not mean healed. It means the body is no longer in immediate danger of collapse. It means the damage has stopped spreading, not that it has been undone. In tetanus, the toxin has already bound to the nervous system by the time the diagnosis is made. The harm is not ongoing in the way an infection continues to spread, but it is not reversible either. The nervous system must repair itself through slow biological processes that cannot be accelerated by medication, reassurance, or determination.

This kind of healing does not respond to encouragement or urgency. It unfolds according to timelines that are indifferent to fear and exhaustion. Nerve endings regenerate when they regenerate. Inhibitory pathways resume function when they are able. No amount of vigilance can make that happen faster, yet absence of vigilance can make it fail.

The long middle is defined by waiting, but not passive waiting.

It is waiting with intention. Waiting with structure. Waiting that requires attention, consistency, and restraint. Care becomes repetitive, and repetition becomes protective. The same checks are performed day after day. The same precautions are maintained long after they stop feeling urgent or intuitive. Small details continue to matter even when the situation feels less dramatic. Progress, when it occurs, is measured in millimetres rather than leaps, and is often recognised only in retrospect, once enough time has passed to reveal what has slowly shifted.

This phase is particularly difficult because it asks for trust without proof.

There are few visible signs that healing is occurring, even when it is. Muscles may remain tight. Swallowing may continue to be unsafe. Fatigue may linger long after the body is no longer in crisis. Setbacks can appear without warning, sometimes triggered by nothing more than normal activity or routine adjustments. All of this can coexist alongside a prognosis that is technically positive, creating a disconnect between what is said and what is felt.

Fear also changes shape during the long middle. It is no longer sharp or urgent. It does not demand immediate action.

Instead, it becomes quieter and heavier, settling into the background of daily life. It surfaces as questions that repeat themselves without resolution. Is this normal. Are we doing enough. Are we missing something. Why is it taking so long. These questions do not arrive as panic. They arrive as persistence.

For owners, this phase can feel lonelier than the initial crisis. Once the immediate danger passes, support often recedes. Friends and family expect improvement. The outside world resumes its usual pace. Concern softens into optimism. Inside the illness, however, life continues to revolve around management, restriction, and watchfulness. The intensity has not disappeared. It has simply become quieter and more sustained.

For the dog, the long middle is not rest. It is work.

The nervous system is relearning how to regulate itself after prolonged disruption. Muscles are relearning how to relax after being locked in contraction. Reflexes are being recalibrated. Sensory thresholds are being reset. None of this occurs evenly or predictably. One function may improve while another stalls. Recovery does not move in straight lines. It circles, pauses, and sometimes slips backward before moving forward again.

This phase is rarely described in detail because it lacks drama. It does not lend itself to clear turning points or tidy conclusions. There are no definitive moments that signal success. And yet, this is the phase where outcomes are shaped. How carefully this period is managed, how consistently precautions are maintained, and how well expectations are understood can determine whether recovery is complete or complicated.

What follows remains with this phase deliberately. It stays inside the waiting, the repetition, and the quiet uncertainty that follows survival. It examines why stabilisation is not the end, why rest becomes active treatment, why feeding becomes fraught, and why fear can persist even as danger recedes. It draws on both lived experience and clinical understanding to make sense of a period that is often minimised or misunderstood.

The chapters ahead are not about rescue. They are about endurance. They are about what happens after survival, when healing becomes slow, uncertain, and deeply personal.

This is the long middle. It is where patience is tested, vigilance is sustained, and recovery is quietly determined, day by day, without spectacle.

Chapter 9

Stabilised Is Not Recovered

The word *stabilised* sounds like safety.

It carries the tone of relief. It suggests ground after freefall, a sense that the body has stopped slipping away from itself. It often arrives at the exact moment when people are most desperate to believe that the worst is behind them, and for that reason alone it can feel like permission to finally exhale.

When a veterinarian says a dog is stabilised, owners frequently hear something more than what is being said. They hear that the danger has passed, that the crisis phase has ended, and that recovery has now begun in earnest. The word lands as reassurance, even when it is not intended that way.

In tetanus, *stabilised* has a far narrower meaning.

It means the body is no longer deteriorating in ways that threaten immediate survival. It means vital functions are being maintained within safe margins. It means the disease has stopped advancing fast enough to outrun medical support. It is an important milestone, but it is not a turning point.

It does not mean the damage has been undone.

Stabilisation is a pause, not a resolution. It is the moment where the body stops losing ground, not the moment where it begins to reclaim it. In tetanus, this distinction matters profoundly, because by the time stabilisation is achieved, the toxin has already done its work. The nervous system has already been altered. What remains is not an active infection racing forward, but a body struggling to recover from what has already occurred.

Neurological injury does not heal on the same timeline as infection or inflammation. The tetanus toxin disrupts inhibitory nerve pathways, effectively removing the signals that tell muscles when to relax. Even once the toxin is neutralised or no longer circulating, those pathways do not immediately resume function. They must be rebuilt, recalibrated, and reintegrated into a system that has been operating without them.

That process takes time, and it happens almost entirely out of sight.

This is why a stabilised dog can still look profoundly unwell. Muscle rigidity may persist. Jaw tension can remain significant. Swallowing may continue to be unsafe. Reflexes may be exaggerated, inconsistent, or unreliable. Fatigue can be extreme, both physical and neurological. None of this contradicts stabilisation. It reflects the reality that neurological recovery lags far behind clinical control.

For owners, this is often where confusion takes hold.

The crisis phase of illness is emotionally overwhelming, but it is also strangely clear. Decisions are urgent. The focus is narrow. There is little room for doubt because there is no time for it. Stabilisation removes that clarity. The immediate threat recedes just enough to make space for questions that have nowhere obvious to go.

If she is stabilised, why does she still look like this?
If things are improving, why is progress so slow?
If treatment is working, why does nothing seem different?

These questions are not signs of mistrust. They are signs of a mismatch between expectation and biological reality.

Stabilisation does not flow smoothly into recovery. It creates a plateau. A long, uneven stretch where the body is being held steady while repair occurs beneath the surface. During this time, improvements are often too subtle to register day to day. Muscle tone may soften by degrees rather than visibly relaxing. A swallow reflex may appear intermittently before becoming reliable. Sleep may deepen long before movement improves. Alertness may return without coordination following suit.

Progress exists, but it rarely announces itself.

More often, it reveals itself only in hindsight, when someone looks back weeks later and realises that what once required constant vigilance has slowly become manageable.

This phase is also where expectations from the outside world begin to clash with lived reality. Friends and family hear the word *stabilised* and assume improvement should now be obvious. Support tapers. Check-ins become less frequent. There is an unspoken sense that things should be moving on, that the illness has entered its closing chapter.

Inside the long middle, nothing feels finished.

Care remains intense. Restrictions remain strict. Vigilance does not ease. The dog still requires protection from overstimulation, careful handling, controlled environments, and constant monitoring. Stabilisation reduces risk, but it does not remove it. The margin for error may be wider than during crisis, but it is still narrow.

Setbacks are common during this phase, and they are often deeply unsettling for owners. A bad day after a good one can feel like regression. A return of stiffness can feel like failure. A new symptom can feel catastrophic. In reality, these fluctuations are expected. Nerve recovery is uneven. Different pathways heal at different rates. Fatigue accumulates. Stress thresholds vary from day to day.

Stabilised does not mean steady.
It means managed.

This is also the point at which the emotional cost of prolonged uncertainty becomes fully visible. The adrenaline of crisis fades, but fear does not disappear. It simply changes shape. It becomes quieter, more persistent, and harder to articulate. It shows up as constant scanning for signs, endless mental comparisons, and a relentless search for reassurance that cannot fully satisfy because there is no definitive marker to point to.

Owners often find themselves living in fractions. Five percent better. Ten percent worse. No change at all. Each small shift feels weighted with significance because there is nothing solid to anchor hope to. Every observation carries meaning because there is no clear finish line in sight.

Veterinary teams understand this phase well, even when it is difficult to convey. They know that stability must be protected aggressively because destabilisation can occur quickly if precautions are relaxed too soon. This is why restrictions remain in place longer than feels intuitive. This is why rest continues to be prescribed even when improvement is anticipated. This is why progress is approached cautiously rather than celebrated prematurely.

The nervous system heals best under conditions of consistency. Predictability reduces demand. Calm reduces firing. Repetition allows pathways to rebuild without interruption. Stabilisation creates the conditions in which recovery can occur, but it does not deliver recovery on a timeline that aligns with human patience or emotional readiness.

Cher's stabilisation did not feel like victory.

It felt like holding.

Holding her body steady. Holding routines in place. Holding fear at bay long enough to continue. There was no moment when everything suddenly turned. There was no clear line between illness and recovery. There was only the gradual recognition, weeks later, that what once felt impossible was slowly becoming manageable.

Stabilisation kept the door open. Recovery still had to make its way through, one careful step at a time.

Chapter 10

Stillness Is Treatment

Stillness feels wrong in almost every way that caring instincts are shaped.

When an animal is unwell, the impulse to act is immediate and powerful. We reach toward touch, toward reassurance, toward movement. We want to coax them back into themselves, to invite them to re-enter the world through play, curiosity, and engagement. Activity feels synonymous with life, and restriction feels like deprivation. Doing nothing feels negligent. Holding back feels cruel.

In tetanus, those instincts must be actively resisted.

Stillness is not the absence of treatment. It is treatment.

The nervous system affected by tetanus is not simply injured. It is overwhelmed. The toxin interferes with the inhibitory signals that normally tell muscles when to relax and sensory systems when to settle. Without those signals, the body remains locked in a state of readiness. Muscles fire too easily.

Reflexes are exaggerated. Sensory input that would normally be filtered or ignored becomes neurologically expensive.

This means that ordinary experiences carry extraordinary cost.

Movement increases neurological demand. Excitement multiplies it. Novelty compounds it further. The nervous system, already struggling to regain control, is pushed repeatedly past its threshold when stimulation is allowed too freely. Stillness, by contrast, reduces demand. It lowers firing. It creates the conditions in which repair can continue without interruption.

This is why rest is prescribed so strictly in tetanus recovery, and why restrictions remain in place long after they feel intuitively necessary. The nervous system cannot heal while it is constantly being asked to respond. It requires long, uninterrupted stretches of low demand. It needs predictability, quiet, and repetition. It needs time spent operating below threshold rather than repeatedly being pushed beyond it.

For Cher, stillness took the form of confinement. She was crated for more than twenty-three hours a day. Even now, that sentence is confronting. It sounds excessive. It sounds punitive. It sounds like something that must surely do harm, especially when applied to a young puppy. But in tetanus recovery, prolonged containment is not punishment. It is protection. The crate became the one environment where her body was safest from itself.

Her mind began to recover long before her nervous system could support it. Mentally, she was alert, curious, responsive. She watched. She listened. She wanted to engage. She wanted interaction, novelty, and movement. Her central nervous system, however, remained fragile, reactive, and easily overwhelmed. That mismatch between mental readiness and neurological capacity is one of the most dangerous phases of tetanus recovery.

The desire to do more does not mean the body can tolerate more. This is where care becomes emotionally difficult.

Holding a dog in stillness when they appear eager and bright feels deeply wrong. Holding a four-month-old puppy in stillness can feel unbearable. Puppies are built for movement. Their learning, confidence, and joy are shaped through exploration, play, and constant physical engagement. Preventing that feels like denying something essential, even when the intention is protective.

Tetanus forces a different priority.

Movement that appears harmless can trigger spasms. Excitement that looks joyful can lead to exhaustion. Overstimulation can undo days of careful progress in minutes. The nervous system, still rebuilding inhibitory control, cannot yet regulate itself in the face of demand. What looks like resilience from the outside may be fragile tolerance underneath.

The crate becomes a boundary the dog cannot yet hold for themselves.

For Cher, stillness was one of the hardest parts of recovery. She wanted to engage long before she could sustain it. She sought interaction, closeness, and stimulation while her body was still unable to cope with the neurological cost of those experiences. Protecting her from her own eagerness required discipline, restraint, and trust in a process that offered no immediate reassurance.

It felt counterintuitive and deeply uncomfortable.

What made it harder was knowing that she did not understand the reason for the boundary. She did not know she was healing. She did not know that restriction was protective. She only knew that she wanted out. Holding that line meant absorbing her frustration without responding to it. It meant not allowing my own discomfort, guilt, or need to soothe to override the plan that was keeping her safe.

Stillness demanded emotional discipline from me, not from her.

This aspect of tetanus care is rarely acknowledged. Treatment plans are often described in clinical terms, but their success depends just as much on the caregiver's ability to tolerate feeling unkind while doing what is necessary. The temptation to loosen restrictions is constant, particularly when the dog looks alert, engaged, and hopeful. It is easy to mistake brightness for readiness.

Interest is not readiness.

For Cher, stillness meant brief, carefully structured periods out of the crate, followed immediately by return to rest. It meant no spontaneous play, no indulgence in excitement, no testing of limits simply to see if she could manage it. The plan remained the plan, even when my instincts urged flexibility.

Especially then.

Stillness is not deprivation. It is the deliberate creation of conditions that allow the nervous system to heal. Every hour spent in calm reduces cumulative fatigue. Every day without neurological overload allows repair to continue uninterrupted. Stillness stacks small gains that are not immediately visible but become meaningful over time.

Progress during this phase is subtle and easily missed. It appears first in rest rather than action. A softer expression during sleep. A jaw that loosens overnight. Muscles that release more fully when the body is still. These are the earliest signs that inhibitory control is slowly returning.

Stillness also protects against setbacks. Fatigue is one of the most underestimated risks in tetanus recovery. The body may appear capable until it suddenly is not. Overexertion can collapse fragile gains and significantly prolong recovery. This is not fragility. It is physiology. A nervous system that is rebuilding cannot tolerate repeated demand without cost.

The nervous system heals through repetition without variation. Each calm day reinforces stability. Each quiet night allows regeneration to continue. Introducing demand too early interrupts that process and resets the clock.

Owners often ask when restrictions can ease.

The answer is not when the dog seems ready.

The answer is when the nervous system demonstrates tolerance without consequence. That proof emerges slowly, through consistency, through the absence of regression, and through stability that holds even when small demands are introduced deliberately and briefly.

Stillness is not doing nothing.

It is doing exactly what the body needs, even when that conflicts with instinct, emotion, and expectation.

In tetanus, healing does not come from encouragement, stimulation, or effort. It comes from restraint applied with intention, patience, and compassion.

Stillness, enforced with care and purpose, is not unkind.
It is lifesaving.

Chapter 11

When Appetite Lies

Eating is supposed to mean safety. It is one of the first signs we reach for when we want reassurance that recovery has begun. Appetite returns, bowls empty, routines resume, and the body appears to remember how to be well. In illness, eating becomes shorthand for improvement, a visible marker that fear can finally loosen its grip.

In tetanus, eating does not offer that reassurance.

It offers risk.

Swallowing is one of the most neurologically complex actions the body performs. It requires precise coordination between the jaw, tongue, throat, and upper airway, all timed perfectly to protect the lungs while allowing nourishment to pass. This coordination depends on inhibitory nerve pathways that tell muscles when to relax as well as when to contract. In tetanus, those inhibitory signals are disrupted. Muscles tighten, but they do not release properly. The sequence that normally keeps food out of the airway breaks down.

A dog may want to eat long before they can swallow safely.

This creates a dangerous mismatch. Appetite can return while swallowing remains compromised. Hunger looks like progress, but in tetanus recovery hunger does not equal readiness. The desire to eat becomes emotionally reassuring and medically concerning at the same time.

Jaw rigidity may persist. The tongue may not move freely. Throat muscles may contract out of sequence. Even a small amount of food or water can slip into the wrong place. Aspiration becomes the central fear, because when food or liquid enters the airway, the consequences can be severe, sudden, and life threatening.

Aspiration pneumonia is one of the most serious complications of tetanus recovery. It does not require a dramatic choking episode. A single unsafe swallow can be enough. It can develop quietly and progress rapidly, particularly in bodies already weakened by prolonged illness.

This is why feeding after tetanus is approached with extraordinary caution.

Texture matters. Consistency matters. Position matters. Timing matters. Environment matters. Feeding becomes structured, deliberate, and clinical rather than intuitive or comforting. Food is softened or fully pureed to reduce effort and risk. Portions are kept small to prevent fatigue. Feeding is slow and carefully paced. Observation does not end when the bowl is empty. It continues through breathing patterns, posture, and recovery afterward.

Hydration is often managed separately because drinking requires a different swallowing pattern and can be even harder to control. Intravenous fluids are frequently used early in recovery to protect the airway while maintaining hydration. In more severe cases, nutritional support is delivered through a feeding tube while the dog remains in intensive care.

For Cher, tube feeding was used during her time in ICU.

The feeding tube allowed calories and hydration to be delivered safely while completely bypassing unsafe swallowing during the most critical phase of her illness. It was not a sign of failure or severity escalation. It was a protective measure, designed to reduce risk while her nervous system was overwhelmed and unstable.

As discharge approached, the question of longer-term nutritional support became unavoidable.

A PEG tube was discussed.

A PEG, or percutaneous endoscopic gastrostomy tube, is a feeding tube placed directly into the stomach through the abdominal wall. It allows nutrition, hydration, and medication to be delivered without using the mouth or throat at all. In tetanus recovery, PEG placement is often the safest option when swallowing remains unreliable or when prolonged nutritional support is required outside the hospital environment.

PEG tubes carry their own risks. Placement requires anaesthesia. Infection at the insertion site is possible. Care and hygiene must be meticulous. Owners must be trained to manage feeds safely at home. However, when swallowing is unsafe, the risks of not placing a PEG can be far greater. Aspiration pneumonia, repeated setbacks, and sudden deterioration are far more dangerous than the controlled risks of tube feeding when it is clinically indicated.

This decision is never taken lightly.

In Cher's case, the decision rested on two factors. Her clinical assessment and my ability to feed her safely at home.

Before discharge, Cher's swallowing was reassessed carefully. While still impaired, it was judged stable enough to allow controlled oral feeding under strict conditions. Just as importantly, my capacity to manage that process safely was evaluated honestly. This was not assumed. It was demonstrated.

Feeding became a diagnostic ritual.

Her food was fully pureed to a liquid consistency. Portions were prepared in the smallest possible amounts. Each mouthful was offered slowly, with her head gently lifted and tilted back to support a safer swallowing angle. I watched every movement of her throat. Every pause. Every breath between swallows. Feeding stopped at the first sign of hesitation, fatigue, tension, or neurological overload.

This was not feeding for satisfaction or fullness. It was feeding for safety.

Based on this combined assessment, the PEG tube was not placed. Cher's ICU feeding tube was removed prior to discharge. Had her swallowing been less stable, or had I not been confident and capable of following a strict feeding protocol, a PEG would have been placed without hesitation.

The decision was not about avoiding intervention. It was about choosing the right one.

But even when tube feeding is temporary, its effects linger. When a dog is fed through a tube, the normal act of eating through the mouth is interrupted. Rituals around food disappear. Hunger remains, but the ability to satisfy it in familiar ways is removed. The drive to eat does not diminish. It intensifies.

This can amplify food related behaviours.

Before tetanus, Cher already carried a history of resource guarding. When she first came to me, we were actively working on teaching her that food was safe, plentiful, and did not need defending. She was learning to share. She was learning calm. Those foundations mattered.

Then tetanus intervened.

Restricted feeding, delayed access, altered routines, and prolonged hunger resurfaced those instincts during recovery. This was not a behavioural failure. It was a predictable response to physiological stress, neurological disruption, and scarcity imposed by medical necessity.

At the same time, Cher was entering a rapid growth phase. She was moving from three months toward four, and her body demanded nourishment at precisely the moment her recovery required limitation. Growth amplifies hunger signals. It creates urgency. Her body asked for more even when safety required restraint.

This tension defined feeding during this phase.

She needed nourishment to grow.
She needed restriction to survive.

Every aspect of feeding became controlled. Size. Texture. Quantity. Speed. Even the way food was delivered mattered. She wanted to scoff. She wanted to gulp. She wanted normality. Instead, she was given measured amounts, slowly, under constant supervision.

Watching a growing puppy want food and not be able to have it freely feels cruel. Denying fullness feels wrong. But overfeeding carried real risk. A swallow taken too quickly, a volume too large, or a moment of fatigue could undo progress and place her lungs in danger.

Resource guarding is not simply a training inconvenience or a phase that resolves on its own. It is a safety issue with real consequences. When a dog learns that access to food is uncertain, restricted, or easily lost, protective behaviours can become instinctive rather than intentional. These behaviours are driven by fear, scarcity, and the nervous system's attempt to secure survival, not by dominance or defiance.

In dogs recovering from serious illness, particularly those who have experienced prolonged hunger and neurological stress, the risk is amplified. A dog startled while eating, interrupted unexpectedly, or approached when already fatigued may react reflexively rather than thoughtfully. Bites that occur in these moments are often sudden and unanticipated.

In family environments, this risk carries additional weight. Children move unpredictably. Other animals do not read subtle stress signals reliably. Well-meaning adults may intervene without recognising warning signs. When resource guarding is ignored, fear can harden into habit.

This is why it must be addressed deliberately.

In Cher's case, those early training foundations mattered. Because calm feeding and sharing had already been introduced before illness, the behaviour did not take permanent hold. With time, consistency, and the gradual return of normal routines, the guarding softened and resolved. She returned to eating alongside Elton.

This mattered for more than harmony. Resource guarding is a preventable safety risk when addressed early and thoughtfully.

Feeding during this phase was never just about calories.

It was about airway protection, neurological healing, behaviour, development, and long-term quality of life. Fear did not disappear. It evolved. In crisis, fear is loud. In feeding, fear becomes quiet and constant. It sits with every meal.
Swallowing returns gradually as nerve pathways regain coordination. Muscles relearn timing. Reflexes stabilise. What was once dangerous becomes manageable, then routine. But that progression cannot be rushed.

Food does not heal tetanus. Time does.

Feeding is about supporting the body, protecting the airway, preserving behaviour, and respecting development while time does its work. When eating becomes safe again, it does not arrive with certainty. It arrives quietly, one calm meal at a time, one uneventful swallow after another, one risk removed rather than ignored.

Until then, caution is not anxiety.
It is wisdom.

Chapter 12

What the Research Quietly Confirms

By the time most people begin searching for research on tetanus, they are already in crisis. This is not curiosity driven reading. It is urgent, emotional, and often undertaken in moments of exhaustion and fear, in hospital waiting rooms, late at night, or while watching a dog who no longer looks like themselves. People search because they want certainty. They want timelines. They want to know what happens next. What they usually encounter instead is ambiguity.

The veterinary literature on canine tetanus is limited. Case numbers are small, studies are retrospective, and conclusions are cautious. Many papers analyse fewer than twenty cases, sometimes collected over many years. Others span decades simply to gather enough data to identify patterns. This scarcity can feel alarming to owners, as though the condition is too rare to understand properly. In reality, it reflects how infrequently tetanus is encountered in companion animal practice rather than a lack of clinical knowledge or effort.

Tetanus is not poorly understood because it is unpredictable. It is poorly studied because it is uncommon. Most veterinarians will never see a confirmed case in their careers. Those who do may encounter it once, often late in its progression and without the benefit of early textbook signs. As a result, the research that exists is built largely on accumulated clinical experience rather than large-controlled trials. When those experiences are examined together, they tell a remarkably consistent story.

The earliest signs of tetanus in dogs are almost universally described as subtle and misleading. Veterinary case series repeatedly document initial presentations involving eye changes, facial tension, jaw stiffness, altered posture, or a dog that appears alert but unable to relax. These signs are frequently misattributed to minor or self-limiting conditions such as conjunctivitis, muscle strain, behavioural changes, or normal puppy development. The literature does not frame this as error or failure. It explains that early tetanus does not resemble a neurological emergency and does not announce itself as a crisis.

By the time classic signs such as generalised rigidity or severe spasms are evident, the disease has often progressed significantly. This delay is not typically the result of poor care, but a direct consequence of how tetanus evolves. The toxin interferes gradually with inhibitory nerve pathways, allowing the body to compensate until it no longer can. Recognition often arrives only when compensation fails.

Research also clarifies one of the most difficult realities for owners to accept. There is no medication that cures tetanus. Antibiotics are recommended to eliminate any remaining *Clostridium tetani* at the site of infection and prevent further toxin production, but they do not reverse neurological damage. Antitoxin can neutralise toxin that is still circulating in the body, but once the toxin has bound to nerve tissue, it cannot be dislodged. At that point, no drug can undo what has already occurred.

This explains why tetanus behaves so differently from most infections. By the time diagnosis is made, the bacteria may no longer be active, yet the disease continues to progress. What drives clinical signs is not infection, but the disruption of inhibitory neurotransmission. Recovery depends on the restoration of these pathways rather than elimination of the original cause.

The literature is explicit about why recovery is slow. Nerve healing is inherently slow. Inhibitory synapses must be rebuilt. Motor neurons must relearn balance and modulation. Muscles that have been held in prolonged contraction must relearn how to release. There is no intervention that meaningfully accelerates this process. Healing unfolds at the pace dictated by biology.

For this reason, supportive care is not an adjunct to treatment. It is the treatment. Veterinary research consistently emphasises that outcomes depend less on a single decisive intervention and more on sustained, meticulous management over time. This includes sedation to control spasms and prevent exhaustion, environmental control to reduce stimulation, careful nutritional support to maintain strength without risking aspiration, respiratory monitoring to detect fatigue early, and ongoing reassessment to adjust care as the disease evolves.

These measures rarely appear dramatic, but they are decisive. Survival depends on maintaining stability long enough for neurological recovery to occur.

The research also confirms that recovery from tetanus is rarely linear. Improvement in one system may coincide with temporary deterioration in another. Facial muscles may relax while gait remains stiff. Swallowing may improve while jaw rigidity persists. Periods of calm may be interrupted by setbacks. These fluctuations are described in the literature as expected features of neurological recalibration rather than signs of treatment failure.

Setbacks are common because tetanus affects multiple systems simultaneously. Continuous muscle contraction increases oxygen demand and fatigue. Prolonged immobility raises the risk of pressure injuries. Swallowing dysfunction increases the likelihood of aspiration pneumonia. Gastrointestinal motility may slow, and secondary infections can develop. This is why prolonged intensive care is recommended for moderate to severe cases whenever it is available, even when outward progress appears minimal.

Clinicians consistently report that the most common question asked by owners is always the same: when will they get better? The research offers no single answer, because none exists. Outcomes are influenced by multiple interacting factors, including the severity of disease at presentation, the speed and timing of intervention, the individual dog's physiology, age, and access to intensive care. Two dogs with outwardly similar signs may recover at entirely different rates. This variability does not reflect failure of treatment or inconsistency in care. It reflects biology.

Importantly, the literature also offers a quiet but significant reassurance. Dogs that survive the acute phase of tetanus and avoid major complications often go on to recover fully. Neurological function can return. Muscle tone can normalise. Behaviour can stabilise. Puppies can resume development. Adult dogs can return to their baseline. These outcomes are possible, but only when the dog is supported long enough for recovery to occur.

The research does not celebrate heroics, dramatic interventions, or quick wins. It does not promise certainty or speed. Instead, it validates patience. It confirms that stillness is not passive, restraint is not neglect, cautious feeding is not fear based, and waiting is not doing nothing. It affirms that tetanus recovery exists in what can only be described as a long middle, a prolonged phase where little appears to change on the surface while everything essential is happening underneath.

Cher's experience did not contradict the research. It followed it closely. What felt uncertain was anticipated. What felt slow was expected. What felt relentless was necessary. The literature does not offer comfort in the way people often want, but it quietly confirms something essential.

When tetanus is recognised, supported, and managed with discipline and care, recovery is possible.

Not because of a single drug or decisive moment.

But because the body is given the time it needs to heal.

That is what the research quietly confirms.

Part IV:

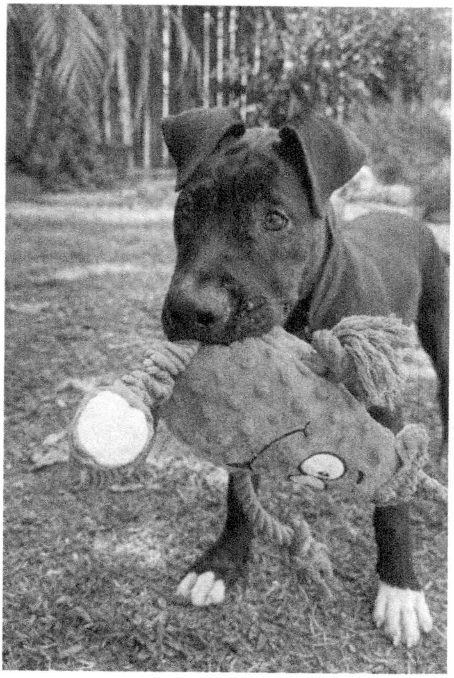

Returning to Life

There is a particular quiet that follows survival, and it is not the quiet people imagine. It is not the hush of machines switching off or alarms falling silent. It is the quieter absence of constant escalation. The needles are no longer being replaced hourly. The intravenous lines are no longer being adjusted and resecured. Feeding tubes are removed. Bandages are reduced. The intensity of intervention eases, not because the body is finished healing, but because it no longer requires moment-by-moment containment. From the outside, this quiet looks like resolution. It looks like recovery has arrived simply because the visible signs of crisis have receded.

In tetanus, this assumption is deeply misleading. The end of the emergency does not mark the end of the illness. It marks a transition into a phase that is less visible, less dramatic, and often more demanding to endure. What disappears is not the disease, but the immediacy of its threat. What remains is a body that must relearn how to function without constant neurological strain, and a nervous system that continues to operate under altered rules long after hospital care has stepped back.

Part IV exists for this stretch of time. It exists for what comes after intensive care, after the drips, the IV access points, the feeding tubes, and the careful restraint that kept the body safe while it could not protect itself. It exists for the return home, where recovery becomes quieter and responsibility becomes heavier. This is the long tail of healing, where progress is no longer overseen by teams and protocols, but held together by consistency, patience, and judgment in the absence of constant reassurance.

This phase is where improvement is real but fragile. The nervous system continues to recalibrate long after medical supervision recedes. Muscles that have lived in contraction remember tension before they remember release. Fatigue appears without warning, not because something is wrong, but because healing itself is metabolically expensive. A dog may look well long before their body feels safe, and that mismatch can be profoundly confusing for everyone involved.

Behavioural and developmental recovery often lag behind physical stability. Movement may return before coordination is reliable. Engagement may appear before the nervous system can tolerate stimulation. What looks like readiness can still conceal vulnerability. This creates a delicate period where outward signs suggest normality while internal systems are still negotiating balance. The danger in this stage is not collapse, but overestimation, the belief that because the body is no longer failing, it is therefore finished healing.

For owners, this phase can feel unexpectedly disorienting. During the crisis, decisions are urgent but clear, guided by expertise, oversight, and constant reassessment. After discharge, that structure dissolves. Support often recedes just as uncertainty reappears in quieter forms. Fear no longer shouts. It settles into constant vigilance. Progress is no longer measured by clinical parameters but by subtle shifts that are easy to doubt and difficult to trust.

Setbacks in this phase feel personal. Without the buffer of hospital care, every change carries weight. A stiff day can feel ominous. Fatigue can feel like regression. Owners find themselves scanning constantly, replaying decisions, questioning whether they are doing too much or not enough.

The emotional labour of recovery often intensifies rather than resolves once the dog comes home.

For dogs, this phase is work. Returning to movement is not just about strength, but about neurological confidence. Returning to play requires coordination that may still be unreliable. Returning to eating normally requires swallowing patterns that must be re-established carefully. Returning to social cues demands emotional regulation that may have been disrupted by prolonged illness, restraint, and separation. The body remembers illness longer than the environment does, and this mismatch can be deeply destabilising.

Recovery in this phase does not move forward in straight lines. It advances, pauses, and occasionally slips backward before progressing again. Some systems recover quickly while others lag behind. One day may feel almost normal, followed by another that feels inexplicably heavy. This variability is not failure. It is the nature of neurological recalibration. The nervous system does not reset all at once. It renegotiates safety gradually, retreating when overstimulated and advancing again when conditions allow.

Part IV explores what recovery actually looks like once the crisis has passed and the work becomes quieter. It examines the residual effects of tetanus on the body and nervous system, the emotional imprint left on both dog and owner, and the practical realities of rebuilding life after prolonged vulnerability. It addresses patience fatigue, lingering hypervigilance, behavioural changes, and the persistent temptation to rush normality simply because survival has already been achieved.

This section is not about vigilance in crisis. It is about wisdom after it. Surviving tetanus is not the end of the story. Learning how to live after it, with respect for what the body has endured and humility about how long healing can take, is where recovery is finally completed.

.

Chapter 13

Bringing Her Body Back

When Cher came home, she did not look better in any way that would have reassured an untrained eye. Her face was still tightly constricted, the muscles around her muzzle and forehead drawn into an expression that did not belong to a puppy. Her eyes continued to roll back intermittently, with the third eyelid appearing far more often than it should. The softness that normally defines a young dog's expression was absent. There was no visual marker that signalled improvement, no moment that announced recovery. What had changed was not her condition, but her location.

Going home creates a powerful illusion of safety. Leaving hospital often carries an unspoken promise that the danger has passed, that the worst is over, and that recovery will now unfold naturally. For many illnesses, this assumption is reasonable. For tetanus, it is not. Discharge does not mean resolution. It means the condition has stabilised enough to be managed without constant medical supervision. The neurological injury remains. The toxin has already done its work. What follows is a long and fragile phase in which deterioration is still possible and setbacks can occur without warning.

That distinction mattered deeply in how Cher's recovery was managed. She came home not because she was well, but because her condition could be monitored, fed, and controlled with a level of discipline that replicated the protective environment of hospital care as closely as possible. There were no longer IV pumps, feeding tubes, or staff rotating through shifts to observe every change. The responsibility for noticing subtle deviation moved entirely with her.

This is where vigilance replaces crisis. The adrenaline of emergency is gone, but the margin for error remains narrow. I did not assume that home meant safe. I understood that the risk had not disappeared, only changed form. Cher was booked into veterinary appointments every week, and sometimes twice a week, not as a reassurance ritual but as active surveillance. The threshold for concern was deliberately low. If her breathing altered, she was seen. If her muscle tension increased, she was seen. If her eyes worsened, she was seen. If anything felt off, she was seen. There was no waiting to see whether things would settle on their own, because tetanus does not reward patience when vigilance is required.

Even routine puppy milestones were treated differently during this phase. Shortly after discharge, Cher lost a puppy tooth. In a healthy puppy, this would barely register. In a dog recovering from tetanus, it mattered. Any break in the gums carried a risk of infection. Any infection carried the potential to destabilise a nervous system still recalibrating after neurological injury. She was examined, and precautionary antibiotics were administered. This was not because there was evidence of infection, but because prevention mattered more than reaction. Tetanus does not tolerate complacency, and recovery does not allow for assumptions.

At the time of discharge, Cher weighed 20.1 kilograms. On paper, this might appear unremarkable or even healthy. In reality, for an American Staffy cross of her size and frame, it reflected interrupted development rather than robustness. Prolonged illness, restricted feeding for safety, and the metabolic cost of neurological injury had slowed her physical growth at a point when her body should have been building rapidly. This is a critical but often misunderstood aspect of recovery in puppies.

Growth does not pause during illness. Developmental signals continue to drive appetite, muscle formation, and skeletal expansion even when the body is unwell. When nourishment is restricted for safety or when the nervous system is under sustained stress, physical development does not stop. It defers. The puppy continues to grow on the inside while the body waits for conditions that allow it to express that growth safely.

Once stability is restored, that deferred growth often arrives quickly and forcefully. In the weeks following discharge, Cher's body began to do what it had been trying to do all along. A rapid growth spurt followed, making clear just how much development had been delayed. In one four-day period alone, she gained four kilograms. By five months of age, she weighed thirty kilograms, a size that finally aligned with her structure, breed mix, and expected trajectory.

Rapid growth, however, introduces its own risks. Growth is metabolically demanding. It requires energy, coordination, and neurological integration. During that growth spurt, there was a day when Cher was noticeably more fatigued than her established tetanus recovery baseline. She was quieter, less resilient, and not bouncing back from rest in the way she had been. She also ran a temperature. In another puppy, this might have been monitored cautiously at home. In a dog recovering from tetanus, it required immediate veterinary assessment.

She was seen. The fatigue and temperature were managed under veterinary oversight, with the understanding that even transient physiological stressors can place additional load on a nervous system still recalibrating. Growth itself can tip a fragile balance. When layered on top of neurological recovery, it must be respected rather than dismissed.

This is why ordinary puppy changes are not ordinary in this context. Teething, growth spurts, minor infections, fatigue, temperature fluctuations, and behavioural shifts all carry amplified significance in a recovering tetanus dog. None of them can be viewed in isolation. Each one interacts with a system that is still learning how to regulate itself, and each one has the potential to push that system beyond its current capacity.

This reality shaped every decision. Movement was limited even as her strength increased. Stimulation was carefully managed even as her confidence returned. Feeding remained precise even as her appetite surged. Eating and drinking were controlled not to deny nourishment, but to deliver it safely. Each restriction served a purpose. Each boundary protected a system still healing beneath visible growth.

Holding this balance was emotionally difficult. Watching a puppy grow rapidly while continuing to impose limits feels counterintuitive. Growth suggests readiness. Energy suggests health. But tetanus recovery does not track neatly alongside physical development. Cher's body was growing faster than her central nervous system could regulate. Restraint was not delaying recovery. It was allowing two competing processes to realign rather than collide.

Bringing her body back to life did not begin with activity. It began with containment. Her instincts were ahead of her physiology. She wanted to play, to run, to wrestle with Elton, to reclaim the world she remembered. But her nervous system could not yet support sustained engagement. Excitement still tipped into tension. Fatigue still arrived abruptly. Muscles tightened before she recognised she needed to stop.

Recovery became an exercise in protection rather than encouragement. Activity was introduced in the smallest possible increments. Short, controlled movements were followed by long periods of rest. Gentle walking replaced free play. Engagement was time limited and deliberate. Progress was measured not by what she could do, but by how well she recovered afterward. If her muscles softened again, activity could continue. If her breathing remained calm, the plan held. If tension escalated, everything stopped. Stillness remained a form of treatment.

Muscles that have been held rigid do not regain flexibility through exertion alone. They relearn relaxation through safety, repetition, and time. The nervous system must experience calm without constant stimulation before movement can be layered back in without reactivating protective tension. Physical rehabilitation after tetanus is not about building strength first. Strength comes later. The early work is about regulation, coordination, and teaching the body that it no longer needs to brace against an invisible threat.

Over time, her recovery became more predictable. Muscles softened more quickly after activity. Fatigue took longer to arrive. Play extended without triggering collapse or tension. These changes were gradual and uneven. Some days felt like progress. Others felt like regression. Neither told the full story. The body does not heal in straight lines.

As weeks passed, movement returned not as bursts, but as rhythm. Walking became smoother. Transitions from rest to activity became less abrupt. Her posture changed. Her face softened. Her body began to support her instincts rather than lag behind them. For a puppy, this process unfolded alongside development. Growth continued. Confidence emerged.

Coordination improved. All of it layered on top of a nervous system still relearning inhibition.

The task was never to accelerate recovery. It was to prevent growth from overwhelming it.

Cher did not recover because she was pushed forward. She recovered because she was protected long enough to carry herself.

That is what bringing her body back to life looked like.

Not revival.
Relearning.

Chapter 14

Re-entering the World Safely

Re-entry does not happen all at once, and it is not a return to what was.

When a dog survives tetanus, the world they step back into is unchanged, but their relationship with it is fundamentally different. Streets still exist. Other dogs still move quickly. Sounds still arrive without warning. What has altered is the dog's capacity to absorb those things without consequence.

The nervous system has been disrupted at a level that is invisible to most observers. There is no wound to point to. No marker on the body that signals fragility. Yet internally, the systems responsible for regulation, inhibition, recovery, and safety are still recalibrating. Sounds, movement, excitement, touch, and novelty are no longer neutral. They carry weight. They demand energy. They must be reintroduced carefully, through a body that is still learning how to regulate itself.

This is where risk quietly reappears.

On the surface, recovery can look convincing. Muscle tone begins to soften. Appetite stabilises. Growth resumes. Energy flickers back to life. For a puppy especially, this creates pressure to normalise quickly. Developmental windows feel urgent. Missed experiences feel permanent. Owners are often told not to "*wrap them in cotton wool,*" to make up for lost time, to get them back to being a dog.

But neurological recovery does not respond to urgency.

It responds to safety.

A nervous system cannot be rushed into regulation. It cannot be trained into resilience. It rebuilds only when the environment repeatedly proves that nothing bad follows stimulation. Safety must be experienced, not explained.

After many weeks of near total crate containment at home, Cher's body had reached a point where cautious re-entry could begin. Her eating was more consistent. Her muscle tension, while still present, had softened enough to suggest that her nervous system was beginning to regain some control. Only then was she allowed her first step back into the outside world.

That step was five minutes.

Five minutes outside, alone. No Elton. No stimulation. No encouragement. No expectation of movement beyond what she chose herself. This was not freedom. It was assessment.

Those first outings were not about enjoyment or enrichment. They were about tolerance. How did her body respond afterward. Did tension increase or resolve. Did fatigue linger beyond what was expected. Did her breathing change. Could she settle again once returned to the crate, or did rest remain elusive. These details mattered more than what happened outside. When these brief, solitary exposures were consistently tolerated, we progressed carefully.

Walking came next.

Four weeks after discharge, our first walk measured 278 metres. It took seventeen minutes. This was not a puppy stopping to sniff. This was a puppy in neurological recovery, placing each step deliberately, conserving energy, managing rigidity beneath the surface. The pace was slow because it had to be. And when the walk ended, it was followed by extended stillness in the crate.

Every exertion was countered with rest.

That was the rule.

Physical effort required recovery time. Mental stimulation required recovery time. Emotional arousal required recovery time. Nothing was allowed to accumulate. Nothing was allowed to compound. Stillness was not the absence of care. It was the mechanism of care.

Only once this rhythm was established did we begin to reintroduce interaction with Elton.

Even then, it was controlled. Both dogs on lead. No running. No jumping. No body contact that could escalate into play. Although Cher's body had softened, an undercurrent of rigidity remained. A Staffy body slam, even a playful one, could have resulted in serious injury or a neurological setback that would not necessarily appear immediately.

Elton understood.

For a two-year-old male Staffy, his restraint was remarkable. He stayed close without demanding engagement. He adjusted his energy. He watched. He waited. It was as though he sensed what she needed and matured into the role she required of him, patiently standing guard while she rebuilt herself. His presence became regulating rather than stimulating.

As Cher passed physical milestones, we deliberately returned to *K9 Aquatics at Coomera*.

This decision was intentional. Hydrotherapy allows exercise to be controlled, measured, and adjusted in real time. Distance and speed can be recorded. Impact is reduced. Muscle engagement can occur without strain. And for a Staffy, water is not just therapeutic, it is motivating. They are known as land seals for a reason.

With Rick at *K9 Aquatics Coomera*, every session prioritised safety over progress. He was patient. He was observant. He worked with me, not ahead of her body. Each visit was assessed not by how much she did, but by how well she recovered afterward. Tolerance mattered more than achievement.

Only after weeks of hydrotherapy that consistently demonstrated recovery without regression did we consider reintroducing daycare.

There are doggy daycares, and then there is *Master of Puppies.*

Set across more than five acres in Southeast Queensland, it offers space, grass, a dam, and freedom of movement that concrete facilities cannot replicate. It is a place dogs love. But love alone does not make something safe.

Before Cher returned, there were conversations. Plans were put in place. Her return to school was structured. She and Elton travelled by bus as usual, but during the day her play was limited, rest was enforced, and she was monitored continuously. I received regular updates throughout the day. Any change in her behaviour was communicated.

What emerged during this phase was something unexpected.

Before tetanus, my dogs interacted more with others than with each other at daycare. After Cher's return, Elton stayed close. He kept her company. He watched. As the weeks passed and her strength and confidence grew, he gradually gave her space. And she took it willingly, rejoining her friends as her body allowed.

This was not a sudden return to life.
It was a layered one.

Re-entering the world after tetanus is not about exposure. It is about controlled reintroduction. Each environment, interaction, and experience is treated as information. How quickly did she recover afterward. Did muscle tone soften or linger. Did excitement resolve into rest, or did tension persist. The answers determined the pace, not the calendar.

There were moments when re-entry went too far. A longer outing. A busier environment. A day with too many variables. These moments were instructive rather than catastrophic. Increased fatigue, subtle rigidity, or delayed recovery signalled the need to step back.

Stepping back was not failure.
It was feedback.

Recovery is not linear, and re-entry is rarely smooth. Progress involves testing boundaries and then retreating from them before harm occurs. The skill lies in recognising the early signs and responding immediately.

For Cher, safety always took precedence over experience.

If an environment could wait, it did.
If an interaction could be postponed, it was.
If stimulation risked destabilising her progress, it was removed.

This was not fear.
It was respect for a nervous system still recalibrating.

Over time, her tolerance increased. Recovery periods shortened. Novelty no longer triggered lingering tension. Engagement began to resolve naturally into rest rather than fatigue. These shifts were subtle, cumulative, and earned.

Re-entry did not restore what had been lost.
It rebuilt what had been interrupted.

And because it was done slowly, deliberately, and without compromise, the world Cher returned to was one she could sustain.

That is what safe re-entry looks like after tetanus.

Not exposure.
Not bravery measured in speed.

But integration, patience, and trust in the long middle between illness and full recovery.

What is less visible in this phase is that re-entry is not only a process for the dog. It is also a recalibration for the person responsible for keeping them safe. After weeks of vigilance, restraint, and constant assessment, confidence does not return all at once. Even as the dog begins to tolerate more, the world remains charged with risk. Every outing is evaluated. Every interaction is monitored. The body may be healing, but the memory of how fragile it once was does not disappear quickly.

This is not anxiety.
It is adaptation.

The human nervous system, much like the dog's, has learned new rules. Where once excitement was encouraged, now caution lives alongside it. Trust must be rebuilt slowly, not because recovery is uncertain, but because experience has taught what happens when signals are missed. Letting go is not a single decision. It is a series of small permissions, granted only when the body continues to prove it can cope.

There is also a biological reason why restraint remains necessary long after outward improvement is visible. Neurological recovery does not restore regulation evenly. Some pathways recover faster than others. A dog may appear strong, alert, and eager while still lacking the internal brakes that allow stimulation to resolve safely. Overexertion does not always cause immediate collapse. It can surface hours later, or the next day, as fatigue, increased muscle tone, or subtle regression.

This delayed response is why re-entry must remain conservative even when progress is evident.

Puppies are particularly vulnerable in this phase. Their nervous systems are not only healing, they are still developing. Growth, learning, and regulation are happening simultaneously. What looks like resilience can mask fragility. What looks like readiness can exceed capacity. When stimulation outpaces regulation, the nervous system responds the only way it can, by tightening, withdrawing, or exhausting itself.

Understanding this reframes restraint.
It is not holding a dog back.
It is preventing overload while capacity catches up.

Setbacks during re-entry are not signs that recovery has stalled. They are signs that the system is still learning its limits. Recognising this allows intervention before harm occurs. It allows stepping back without shame. It allows progress to continue without punishment.

And then, often quietly, something shifts.
Not a milestone.
Not a dramatic moment.

But a subtle change in how the dog moves through the world. Stimulation no longer lingers in the body. Engagement resolves into rest without effort. Confidence appears without tension underneath it. Recovery stops feeling like management and begins to feel like life again.

When that moment comes, it does not announce itself.
It is noticed in retrospect.

In the absence of vigilance.
In the ease of settling.
In the quiet certainty that the body is no longer fighting itself.

Re-entry, done properly, does not rush toward this moment. It creates the conditions for it to arrive on its own.

That is what safe re-entry looks like after tetanus.
Not exposure.
Not urgency.

But integration, patience, and trust in the long middle between illness and full recovery.

Cher's Key Principles for Safe Re-entry After Tetanus

These principles emerged through trial, observation, and restraint during Cher's recovery.

1. Re-entry is neurological, not behavioural

A dog may look physically improved while still lacking the neurological regulation required to process stimulation safely. Readiness cannot be judged by enthusiasm, energy, or outward appearance alone.

2. Safety must come before exposure

New environments, interactions, and activities should only be introduced when the nervous system can reliably return to baseline afterward. Exposure without recovery increases risk, even when it appears tolerated in the moment.

3. Tolerance matters more than achievement

Progress is measured by how well the dog recovers after an activity, not by how much they can do during it. Delayed fatigue, lingering muscle tension, or difficulty settling are signals to slow down.

4. **Stillness is an active intervention**

Rest is not passive. Stillness allows neurological systems to integrate stimulation and recalibrate. Every physical, mental, and emotional effort must be balanced with sufficient recovery time.

5. **Introduce one variable at a time**

Re-entry should add only one new demand per exposure. Layering novelty, movement, social interaction, and excitement increases the likelihood of overload and delayed regression.

6. **Setbacks are feedback, not failure**

Periods of increased fatigue, rigidity, or delayed recovery indicate that capacity has been exceeded. Responding early by reducing stimulation prevents escalation and protects long-term progress.

7. **The calendar does not determine readiness**

Timelines are unreliable. Neurological recovery progresses unevenly, particularly in puppies whose systems are still developing. The dog's response, not the date, determines pace.

8. **Human vigilance is part of recovery**

The caregiver's ongoing assessment, restraint, and advocacy remain essential long after outward improvement appears. This is not anxiety. It is an adaptive response learned through experience.

9. **Integration, not normalisation, is the goal**

Safe re-entry rebuilds a sustainable relationship with the world rather than forcing a return to pre-illness behaviour. True recovery is indicated by ease, not endurance.

Red Flags During Re-entry

Signs that stimulation has exceeded neurological capacity and re-entry needs to slow.

- **Delayed fatigue**

The dog appears fine during or immediately after an activity but becomes withdrawn, flat, or unusually tired hours later or the following day.

- **Lingering or increased muscle tension**

Rigidity that does not resolve with rest, or stiffness that reappears after exertion, particularly in the jaw, neck, or limbs.

- **Difficulty settling after stimulation**

Restlessness, inability to relax, disrupted sleep, or prolonged agitation following outings or interaction.

- **Changes in breathing or posture**

Shallow, rapid breathing at rest, altered gait, guarded movement, or reluctance to lie down comfortably.

- **Reduced tolerance for touch or interaction**

Subtle withdrawal, irritability, flinching, or avoidance that was not previously present.

- **Regression in skills or confidence**

Loss of previously regained abilities, increased hesitation, or renewed sensitivity to sounds, movement, or novelty.

- **Heightened reactivity without clear cause**

Startle responses, tension, or emotional escalation disproportionate to the stimulus.

- **Recovery taking longer than expected**

Extended rest periods needed to return to baseline, even after low-level activity.

Part V:

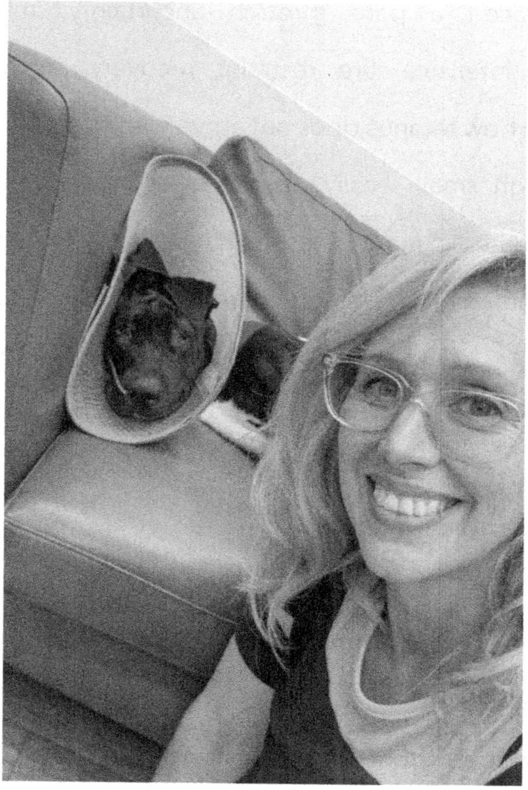

What Every Dog Owner Needs To Know

Up to this point, this book has been Cher's story.

It has traced a path through uncertainty, misdirection, diagnosis, intensive care, restraint, recovery, and re-entry. It has shown how tetanus does not arrive with spectacle or clarity, but through small, easily dismissed changes and decisions made repeatedly under pressure. It has also shown that survival is rarely the result of a single intervention, but of consistency, patience, and the willingness to keep looking when answers are not yet clear.

This final section turns outward.

Not because every dog will experience tetanus, but because every dog owner will one day encounter a moment when something feels wrong and there is no obvious explanation. A shift in behaviour. A change in movement. A look in the eyes that does not quite fit. These moments are common. What is uncommon is knowing how to respond when reassurance arrives faster than resolution.

These chapters are not written to alarm or to overwhelm. They exist to sharpen awareness, validate instinct, and shorten the distance between concern and appropriate care.

Dog owners are not diagnosticians. They are not expected to recognise rare diseases or interpret clinical signs in isolation. But they are the first observers. They see their dogs across contexts and time. They notice the subtle shifts that do not yet meet diagnostic thresholds. They hold the baseline that no textbook, flowchart, or consultation can fully capture.

That position matters more than is often acknowledged.

Too often, early signs are dismissed because they are quiet. Because they do not yet fit a pattern. Because they are inconvenient to explain or easy to rationalise away. This section exists to counter that tendency, not by elevating fear, but by honouring observation.

I have walked through the fire. I have sat in the silence. And now, I stand in a space of clarity, conviction, and contribution.

What follows is written from that place, not as instruction, but as synthesis.

These chapters bring together lived experience, clinical understanding, and what the research quietly confirms. They focus on recognising early warning signs that owners often see first, understanding what truly helps and what unintentionally causes harm, knowing when to insist on further help without guilt or apology, and holding realistic expectations when recovery does not follow a neat or linear timeline.

This is not a checklist, and it is not a rulebook. It does not promise certainty.

What it offers instead is orientation.

A way to make sense of what feels uncertain. A framework for noticing without catastrophising. Language for advocating without escalating. And permission to trust observation when proof has not yet arrived.

If this book can shorten the time between a first uneasy feeling and meaningful intervention for even one dog, then Cher's story reaches beyond her. It becomes a contribution rather than a record.

That is the purpose of this part.

Chapter 15

Early Warning Signs Owners See First

The earliest signs of tetanus in dogs rarely resemble what people expect a neurological emergency to look like. They do not arrive with urgency or spectacle, and they do not announce themselves as danger. Instead, they emerge quietly and often incrementally, as small deviations from normal that appear reasonable when considered individually and easy to dismiss when viewed in context. This is one of the central reasons canine tetanus is so frequently missed in its early stages. It is not due to neglect or incompetence, but because the disease presents itself as normal variation until the accumulating pattern becomes impossible to ignore.

In Cher's case, the early warning signs only became clear after the diagnosis was made. At the time, each sign stood alone and carried a plausible explanation. None appeared serious enough to justify alarm. It was only later, when these observations were placed side by side, that the pattern became visible. This reliance on hindsight is not unusual. Veterinary literature consistently describes the prodromal phase of tetanus as subtle, nonspecific, and highly variable between patients. Owners frequently sense that something is not right long before they can articulate what that something is, because early changes are felt more clearly than they are defined.

One of the first changes I noticed in Cher was in her face. There was no swelling, redness, or obvious injury. What changed was the tension. The muscles across her forehead no longer softened when she rested. Her expression appeared fixed, almost strained, as though she were holding effort without release. Her ears, which normally sat relaxed and expressive, began to draw closer together at the top of her head, held in a position that suggested muscular engagement rather than alertness. Over time, her face appeared subtly gaunt, not from weight loss, but from continuous muscle contraction.

These changes were not dramatic to an unfamiliar observer, but to someone who knew her baseline intimately, they were unmistakable. Veterinary descriptions of early tetanus often refer to facial muscle rigidity and altered cranial nerve involvement, yet these signs rarely appear as obvious spasm in the early stages. Instead, they present as persistent tension and reduced relaxation, which are easily overlooked unless the observer is attuned to what is normal for that individual dog.

Her eyes were the earliest sign that caused unease before I understood why. They did not rest properly. She blinked less frequently, and when she was tired her eyes did not soften into sleep but remained alert and strained. Over time, I observed intermittent upward rolling of the eyes, particularly when she was fatigued, and the third eyelid became intermittently visible. At times this affected one eye, at other times both.

Such signs are commonly attributed to irritation, conjunctivitis, or environmental exposure, and in many cases those explanations are appropriate. However, the tetanus literature notes that early ocular involvement may include altered eye position, reduced blink reflex, and third eyelid protrusion caused by imbalance in muscle tone. In the early stages these signs often fluctuate, appearing and resolving temporarily, which makes them easier to dismiss until persistence forces reconsideration.

Another early change involved Cher's water intake. She began drinking more frequently, not excessively and not urgently, but enough to be noticeable. In a growing puppy, increased thirst is readily attributed to activity levels, weather, diet, or growth.

Yet sustained muscle contraction increases metabolic demand and heat production even before overt rigidity becomes visible. The body compensates quietly at first, and increased hydration can be an early physiological response. This change rarely signals neurological disease on its own, but when viewed alongside muscle tension, fatigue, and altered behaviour, it becomes part of a broader pattern that only makes sense in retrospect.

Cher's movement also changed, though not in a way that suggested weakness or incoordination. She did not stumble or fall. Instead, her movements became careful and deliberate. Tasks that should have been effortless for a puppy her age appeared to require concentration and effort. Play tired her quickly, and excitement drained her rather than energising her. When she lay down, her body did not fully relax, and when she slept, her muscles remained partially engaged.

Veterinary case reports describe this early stiffness as one of the most frequently overlooked signs of tetanus, largely because it lacks the dramatic spasms commonly associated with the disease. The tetanus toxin interferes with inhibitory neurotransmitters, preventing muscles from receiving signals to relax. Early in the disease process, this manifests as continuous low-level contraction rather than obvious rigidity, allowing the condition to progress quietly.

There was also a sound that drew my attention. It was a brief, intermittent snort that appeared without a clear trigger. Dogs make noises, and puppies experiment with their bodies, which makes such sounds easy to dismiss. However, the persistence of this sound placed it in the category of something that did not quite fit. Changes in vocalisation, breathing sounds, or subtle respiratory noises are documented in early tetanus cases and reflect increased reflex sensitivity and altered muscle control. In isolation, these sounds are rarely alarming, but as part of an accumulating picture, they warrant attention.

Behaviourally, Cher remained gentle, responsive, and engaged, yet she was never fully at ease. Her body carried constant tension, as though she were bracing against something unseen. She struggled to sink into rest and appeared unable to fully relax. This kind of unease is often interpreted as anxiety, overstimulation, or temperament. The literature suggests, however, that it more accurately reflects central nervous system overactivation rather than emotional distress. Owners experience it emotionally because that is how it presents, but its origin is neurological.

Veterinary literature describes a range of additional early warning signs that were not all present in Cher. These include jaw stiffness, reluctance to chew, difficulty opening the mouth fully, changes in bark or vocalisation, exaggerated responses to noise or touch, heightened startle reflex, and increased sensitivity to light or sound. Some dogs appear intermittently improved, only to worsen again later. This fluctuation is one of the most misleading features of early tetanus and contributes significantly to delayed recognition.

What makes these early signs particularly dangerous is not their subtlety, but their plausibility. Each sign appears reasonable when considered alone. Tired eyes may be attributed to allergies. Stiff movement may be explained by growth or minor soreness. Increased thirst may be dismissed as heat or activity. Behavioural changes may be framed as mood or

developmental variation. None of these explanations are sufficiently incorrect to demand immediate challenge.
The difficulty arises through accumulation.

As small changes persist, evolve, or begin to overlap, the underlying threat gradually becomes visible. By the time this pattern is recognised, valuable time may have passed. This delay is not a failure of care. It is a structural feature of how early tetanus presents and why the disease so often progresses before it is identified.

This chapter exists to name what is usually unnamed. It validates the instinct that notices when a dog's ears sit differently, when their eyes no longer rest, and when their body appears to be working harder than it should. Veterinary medicine relies on pattern recognition, but owners are the ones who supply the pattern. They observe across time, environment, and behaviour in ways that clinical encounters cannot replicate. The research supports this role more strongly than it is often acknowledged. Early diagnosis of tetanus is associated less with certainty or specialist expertise than with persistence, repeated assessment, and owner advocacy.

It is important to state clearly that the signs described in this chapter do not represent the full range of early presentations of tetanus. No single dog will display all early warning signs, and many will show only a few. The absence of a particular symptom does not rule the disease out. This variability is one of the reasons tetanus remains so difficult to recognise early, even for experienced clinicians.

Veterinary case reports also describe intermittent limb stiffness that resolves with rest, reluctance to climb stairs or jump despite preserved strength, subtle changes in posture such as rigid neck carriage or altered tail position, transient tremors during excitement or handling, difficulty settling despite appearing physically well, mild constipation reflecting early autonomic involvement, hypersalivation, and altered breathing patterns during sleep. These signs are easily attributed to benign causes, particularly in young or active dogs, yet they appear repeatedly in descriptions of early disease progression.

What unites these early signs is not their severity, but their inconsistency. They fluctuate. They overlap with normal variation. They resolve temporarily and then return. This pattern of appearance and disappearance is repeatedly cited in the literature as a contributing factor to delayed diagnosis. Periods of apparent improvement provide reassurance, even as the underlying neurological disruption continues to advance.

For this reason, the most reliable early indicator of tetanus is not a specific symptom, but a pattern that does not settle. A collection of small changes that persist or accumulate without a unifying explanation deserves attention, even when each element appears benign in isolation. Cher did not experience every sign described here, and many dogs will not. Recognising that tetanus rarely presents the same way twice is essential to understanding why early detection depends so heavily on vigilance, familiarity, and trust in observation rather than certainty.

This chapter does not attempt to catalogue every possible early sign of tetanus. The disease does not follow a fixed script, and no list can capture the full range of its early manifestations. What matters most is not the presence or absence of any single symptom, but the pattern that forms when small changes accumulate without resolution. Tetanus announces itself through inconsistency rather than clarity, through fluctuation rather than progression, and through a quiet persistence that resists easy explanation.

The nervous system does not fail all at once. It destabilises gradually, compensating until it no longer can. Survival often begins with permission to trust that something small matters.

Chapter 16

What Helps and What Hurts

When something feels wrong with a dog, most owners respond in ways they have been taught to trust. They observe. They wait. They reassure themselves that time will clarify what is happening. Often, this instinct is rewarded. Many minor issues resolve on their own. Puppies grow. Muscles ache. Eyes become irritated. Behaviour fluctuates. In most situations, waiting is reasonable and appropriate.

In tetanus, waiting is rarely neutral.

What helps in the early stages of tetanus is not decisiveness or certainty. It is persistence. It is the willingness to return when something does not improve and to remain engaged when reassurance does not align with what continues to be observed. A symptom that remains unexplained is not the same as a symptom that is benign. Owners who help their dogs most effectively are not those who panic, but those who do not disengage when the explanation offered fails to account for what they continue to see.

One of the most helpful actions an owner can take is to document change. This does not require clinical language or medical expertise. It requires clarity and consistency. Noting when a sign first appeared, whether it is worsening or fluctuating, and whether it resolves fully between episodes provides information that memory alone cannot reliably supply. Tetanus often advances slowly enough that change feels imperceptible day to day, yet becomes obvious when viewed over a longer span. Documentation allows patterns to emerge that might otherwise remain invisible.

Repeated assessment is another factor that helps. Returning to a veterinarian when a treatment does not produce the expected result is not a challenge to competence. It is an essential part of responsible care. Tetanus is rarely diagnosed at the first visit because its early signs overlap with many far more common conditions. What matters is not immediate accuracy, but recognising when the initial explanation no longer fits the evolving picture. Owners who persist and say that a problem has not settled create the conditions for reassessment. That reassessment is often the turning point.

Clear communication also plays a critical role. Owners who can describe what has changed, rather than what they fear, are more likely to be heard and understood. Statements such as "her eyes do not rest the way they used to," "she seems unable to fully relax," or "she is drinking more and tiring more quickly" convey observable shifts rather than conclusions. These observations may feel subjective, but when taken together they are clinically meaningful. Veterinary medicine relies on pattern recognition, and owners are the primary source of longitudinal pattern data.

Context also matters. Recent wounds, even very small ones, exposure to soil or mud, contact with livestock environments, stagnant water, recent teething or oral injury, growth spurts, immune stress, or concurrent illness all alter risk. None of these factors diagnose tetanus on their own, but they widen the diagnostic frame. When owners share context alongside symptoms, they help clinicians consider possibilities that might otherwise remain peripheral.

Environmental management is another quietly protective factor. Reducing stimulation, limiting handling, and controlling activity can significantly influence symptom expression even before a diagnosis is made. In tetanus, noise, excitement, touch, and exertion can all amplify reflex activity and muscle contraction. Owners who instinctively create calm, low stimulation environments are often providing neurological support without realising it. This restraint is not indulgence or overprotection. It is regulation support for a nervous system under strain.

Access also matters, though it is rarely discussed openly. Access to follow-up appointments, access to referral pathways, and access to emergency or specialist care when uncertainty persists all shape outcomes. Tetanus progression is influenced not only by disease severity, but by how quickly escalation is possible when first-line explanations fail. Owners who ask about next steps early preserve time. In tetanus, time is often more valuable than certainty.

What hurts, by contrast, is dismissal that leads to delay. This dismissal is rarely malicious. It often takes the form of reassurance layered upon reassurance, each reasonable in isolation. Suggestions to wait a few more days, reminders that the dog is still eating or still playful, or assumptions that symptoms are simply developmental can all be accurate and still harmful when they prevent escalation in the face of persistence.

Over-interpreting improvement can also cause harm. Tetanus is characterised by fluctuation. A dog may appear better one day and worse the next. Muscle tone may soften temporarily. Eye signs may recede. Energy may briefly return. These oscillations can create false confidence that the problem is resolving, particularly when apparent improvement coincides with treatment initiation. Both owners and clinicians can be misled by this pattern, mistaking coincidence for response while the underlying disease continues to progress.

Excessive stimulation once concern has been raised is another harmful factor. Repeated handling, unnecessary travel, exposure to busy environments, and attempts to test a dog's limits increase demand on a nervous system that is already struggling to regulate itself. In tetanus, stimulation does not build resilience. It compounds instability.

Well-meaning advice can also cause harm when it encourages normalisation over observation. Suggestions to wait until a dog collapses or deteriorates dramatically reflect a misunderstanding of how tetanus progresses. Collapse is not an early sign. By the time it occurs, the disease is already advanced. Early tetanus requires attention long before dramatic deterioration appears.

Comparison is another quietly damaging influence. Hearing that other dogs behave similarly or that a comparable situation resolved on its own can undermine an owner's confidence in their own observations. Tetanus does not unfold according to averages. It progresses within individual bodies, shaped by exposure, physiology, and timing. Comparison reassures socially, but obscures biological reality.

Perhaps the most damaging factor is self-doubt. Owners who sense something is wrong often talk themselves out of that awareness, particularly when external reassurance conflicts with internal unease. This erosion of confidence delays action. Tetanus exploits delay. Owners who help most effectively are not those who recognise tetanus immediately, but those who trust themselves enough to continue asking questions when answers fail to satisfy.

Cher's outcome was shaped not by a single decision, but by a sequence of choices that favoured persistence over reassurance. She was returned for reassessment when treatment failed to produce improvement. Her symptoms were not accepted as static. Her environment was controlled. Her activity was limited. Her care escalated when uncertainty remained. None of these choices were dramatic. All of them mattered.

What helps in tetanus is not heroics. It is steadiness. What hurts is not ignorance. It is delay disguised as reassurance.

This chapter is not about blame. It is about leverage. Small decisions, repeated consistently, can alter the trajectory of a disease that relies on time and invisibility to advance. Owners do not need to know everything. They need to know when not to disengage.

The next chapter explores what happens when persistence must become insistence, and when reassurance is no longer sufficient.

Chapter 17

When to Insist on Help

Knowing when to insist on help is one of the most underestimated responsibilities of animal guardianship. It is rarely framed as a skill, yet it is one of the most consequential decisions an owner will ever make. Animals do not escalate care for themselves. They do not seek second opinions, request referrals, or question reassurances that do not fully account for what is happening. They rely entirely on the human who knows them best to notice, interpret, and act. This responsibility does not begin at crisis. It begins the moment something feels unresolved.

Many owners hesitate to insist on further assessment because hesitation is often rewarded socially. We are conditioned to be polite, patient, and trusting. We are encouraged to accept reassurance, avoid appearing difficult, and give situations time to resolve. In veterinary settings, where professionals manage heavy caseloads and work within uncertainty, this social conditioning can inadvertently delay escalation. An explanation may sound reasonable. An animal may still be eating. Improvement may appear briefly and then fade. Under these conditions, insisting on help can feel uncomfortable, even when it is motivated by care rather than distrust.

Insistence, however, is not aggression. It is persistence. It is the decision to remain engaged when clarity has not yet arrived.

There are moments when waiting is appropriate and moments when waiting becomes dangerous. The distinction is not always obvious, which is why insistence must be grounded not in panic, but in pattern recognition. When signs persist without resolution, when explanations multiply without converging, when symptoms fluctuate rather than settle, or when an animal's baseline continues to drift, escalation is justified. Asking for further investigation, referral, or monitoring is not a challenge to expertise. It is an extension of the diagnostic process itself.

In animal health and welfare, insistence is often the difference between stabilisation and deterioration. Many serious conditions do not declare themselves clearly at the outset. Neurological compromise, pain syndromes, internal infections, endocrine disorders, and physical illness expressed through behavioural change frequently present in ambiguous ways. Animals compensate. Bodies adapt. Symptoms may hide, soften, or temporarily recede. In these situations, insistence is not about knowing the diagnosis. It is about recognising that uncertainty remains and choosing not to disengage while it does.

Guardians are accountable for the health, safety, and wellbeing of the animals in their care in a way no one else is. That accountability does not transfer when an appointment ends or a provisional explanation is given. It remains continuous. Guardians observe their animals at rest, under stress, during recovery, and across time. Clinicians see snapshots. Owners see trajectories. Both perspectives are valuable, but only one is constant.

One of the most dangerous substitutes for advocacy in modern animal care is crowdsourced certainty, particularly through social media forums and online groups. While these spaces are often well intentioned and emotionally supportive, they are structurally incapable of providing safe medical or behavioural guidance. They do not know your dog. They do not know their full medical history, developmental stage, genetics, prior injuries, vaccination status, neurological baseline, environment, diet, stressors, or training history. They cannot observe subtle changes in posture, movement, eye position, or muscle tone across days and weeks. They do not carry responsibility for outcomes.

Advice offered in these spaces is almost always based on partial information, personal anecdote, breed generalisation, or what worked once under entirely different circumstances. This creates a false sense of reassurance that can delay proper assessment, normalise concerning signs, or encourage inappropriate intervention. Behavioural advice can obscure pain. Medical reassurance can postpone escalation. Confident voices can overwhelm quieter instincts. In the context of serious illness or neurological compromise, such delay is not neutral.

Advocacy does not mean seeking consensus from strangers. It means recognising that visibility, accountability, and continuity of care matter more than volume of opinion. Social media can provide community and empathy, but it cannot replace clinical assessment, longitudinal observation, or decision-making grounded in the full reality of an individual animal's life. When advice feels comforting but discourages further investigation, minimises unresolved change, or encourages waiting despite persistence, it becomes a risk rather than a resource.

Support is not the same as guidance.

Insisting on help also requires recognising when reassurance is insufficient. If something feels wrong and continues to feel wrong, that perception deserves weight. Animals communicate discomfort and dysfunction subtly. They rely on humans to interpret those signals without demanding certainty as a prerequisite for action. Advocacy often begins before evidence becomes definitive. It begins with attention and is sustained through follow-through.

This responsibility extends beyond overt illness. Behavioural changes, withdrawal, aggression, fear responses, altered appetite, disrupted sleep, or changes in interaction patterns all warrant consideration beyond surface explanations. Behaviour is communication. Pain frequently hides behind temperament labels. Stress is often mistaken for disobedience. When behavioural guidance does not account for possible physical causes, insisting on medical assessment is an act of protection rather than overreaction.

Insistence may take many forms. It may involve requesting referral, asking for further diagnostics, returning sooner than suggested, or declining to accept a wait and see approach when nothing has settled. It may involve changing providers when communication breaks down or when concerns are repeatedly minimised. None of these actions require justification beyond unresolved concern.

This is not about distrusting professionals. It is about recognising that medicine is iterative and that guardianship includes the responsibility to remain engaged in that process. Most veterinarians value persistent, observant owners because those owners improve outcomes. They supply information no test can replicate, including time, context, and continuity.

If you are an animal's guardian, you are their first advocate and often their only one. No one else carries that role in full. Advocacy is not about knowing the answer. It is about refusing to disengage when the answer remains unclear. It is about staying present, asking again, and holding attention when something does not sit right.

Animals do not need perfect decisions. They need committed ones.

Insisting on help is not a failure of trust. It is an expression of care.

Chapter 18

Recovery Timelines and Expectations

Recovery from tetanus does not begin when a dog leaves hospital. It begins when the immediate threat to life has passed and the prolonged work of neurological repair takes over. This distinction matters because discharge is often misunderstood as resolution. In tetanus, discharge represents a transition rather than an endpoint. It marks the transfer of responsibility from intensive clinical oversight to sustained care carried out in the home.

Not all dogs survive tetanus. This must be stated plainly. Even with early intervention, intensive care, and appropriate treatment, tetanus remains a life-threatening disease with a significant mortality rate. Dogs may succumb during the acute phase due to respiratory compromise, aspiration pneumonia, autonomic instability, or overwhelming muscle rigidity. Others may survive intensive care only to deteriorate later, when fatigue, infection, or neurological overload exceeds what their bodies can compensate for. Survival is never guaranteed, and recovery is never owed.

For dogs who do survive, recovery is not a return to health so much as a gradual rebuilding of function. The primary injury in tetanus occurs within the central nervous system. The toxin interferes with inhibitory neurotransmission, leaving muscles in a state of persistent activation. Healing depends on the regeneration of nerve terminals and the slow restoration of balance between excitation and inhibition. This process cannot be accelerated. Neural repair occurs unevenly and at different rates across the body. Some pathways recover sooner, while others lag behind. This uneven progression explains why improvement appears inconsistent and why recovery timelines vary so widely between dogs.

There is no universal recovery window. Some dogs show meaningful improvement within weeks, while others require many months before approaching their previous baseline. Puppies may benefit from greater neuroplasticity, yet they face additional strain from growth, developmental demands, and rapidly changing physiology occurring alongside recovery. Adult dogs may stabilise more predictably but often take longer to regain flexibility, coordination, and endurance. Disease severity, duration of toxin exposure, speed of diagnosis, access to intensive care, and avoidance of secondary complications all influence outcome. Two dogs with similar clinical presentations may follow entirely different recovery trajectories.

Discharge from hospital marks a critical shift in responsibility that is frequently underestimated. The most demanding phase of recovery typically unfolds not under continuous veterinary supervision, but in the home, sustained day after day by the caregiver. This phase is labour-intensive, repetitive, and unrelenting. It requires vigilance rather than intervention and consistency rather than action.

Crate containment is often necessary for weeks or months after discharge. This measure is protective rather than punitive. A nervous system in recovery cannot tolerate unregulated movement, excitement, or play without risk of setback. What is less often acknowledged is that crate rest is not passive care. It is an active management process that shapes every aspect of daily life, from feeding and hydration to toileting and temperature control.

Environmental regulation becomes part of treatment. Temperature management is particularly important, especially in warm or humid climates. Dogs recovering from tetanus already operate under increased metabolic demand due to sustained muscle contraction. At the same time, sedation, weakness, and limited mobility reduce their ability to reposition, cool themselves, or signal distress. Poor ventilation, retained heat, or assumptions about comfort can quickly create risk. Bedding must allow airflow. Ambient temperature must be monitored rather than assumed. These are safety requirements, not comfort preferences.

Hydration also becomes an active responsibility rather than a passive provision. A dog recovering from tetanus cannot safely self-regulate fluid intake. Swallowing may remain impaired. Jaw and throat muscles may lack coordination. Fatigue can interrupt drinking. For Cher, water had to be offered deliberately, under close supervision, and in controlled amounts. Each swallow required observation. The task was not simply to provide access to water, but to ensure hydration without aspiration or drowning. Even basic physiological needs required careful management.

Toileting must be structured and controlled. Dogs cannot be allowed to wander or stimulate themselves simply because they need to relieve themselves. They must be taken out on lead, often frequently and briefly, with the sole aim of function rather than enrichment. These outings are not walks. They are controlled tasks followed immediately by a return to stillness. In warm conditions, timing becomes critical to limit heat exposure and exertion that could destabilise recovery.

Medication adherence becomes non-negotiable during this phase. Missed doses matter. Timing matters. Sedatives, muscle relaxants, antibiotics, and adjunct medications do not cure tetanus, but they protect the nervous system while healing occurs. Inconsistent administration increases the risk of breakthrough rigidity, exhaustion, and regression. After discharge, the caregiver becomes the final link in a complex treatment chain. The chain holds only if each link performs reliably.

What is rarely acknowledged in clinical discussions is the emotional toll this stage places on the caregiver. Recovery from tetanus unfolds over weeks or months without a defined endpoint. There is no clear marker that signals when vigilance can safely ease. Care routines must be integrated into daily life alongside work, family responsibilities, and existing demands. Sleep is often fragmented. Decision fatigue accumulates. Hypervigilance becomes a sustained state rather than a temporary response. This cognitive and emotional load is real, even if it remains largely invisible.

There is also a financial reality associated with prolonged recovery. Prescription veterinary diets are often required to support safe swallowing, digestion, and nutritional needs during healing. These diets are significantly more expensive than standard food and may be required for extended periods. Ongoing veterinary reviews, medications, environmental controls, mobility supports, and follow-up investigations add further cost. Even with insurance, out-of-pocket expenses continue. Recovery is measured not only in time and effort, but in sustained financial commitment.

Progress during this phase is rarely dramatic. It is measured in tolerance rather than milestones. A dog may manage a brief increase in activity one week and regress the next due to fatigue, growth, or environmental stress. Periods of apparent stability may be followed by transient stiffness, altered behaviour, or changes in temperature regulation. These fluctuations do not indicate failure. They reflect a nervous system operating near its current capacity.

The emotional impact of this uncertainty compounds over time. Caregivers continually reassess decisions, recalibrate expectations, and question their own judgment. Confidence erodes before it rebuilds. Trust returns slowly, only as the dog's body demonstrates consistency over time. Emotional recovery runs alongside physical healing and often lags behind it.

The most important expectation to release is the idea that recovery follows a shared script. There is no average dog and no standard timeline. There is no correct pace. There is only the individual animal, the nervous system they inhabit, and the care they receive consistently over time.

For dogs who survive and are protected through this prolonged middle phase, the outlook can be cautiously hopeful. Neurological function can return. Muscle tone can normalise. Behaviour can stabilise. Puppies can resume development. Adult dogs can regain quality of life. These outcomes are conditional. They depend on time, restraint, environmental control, financial capacity, and sustained consistency long after urgency fades.

Recovery from tetanus is not marked by a single moment of success. It is confirmed quietly over months, as the nervous system relearns inhibition and the body reclaims balance. Discharge is not the end of treatment. It is the point at which treatment becomes shared responsibility, carried home and sustained by the person who continues to show up without certainty, recognition, or a finish line.

Understanding this does not make recovery easier. It makes it honest.

Part VI:

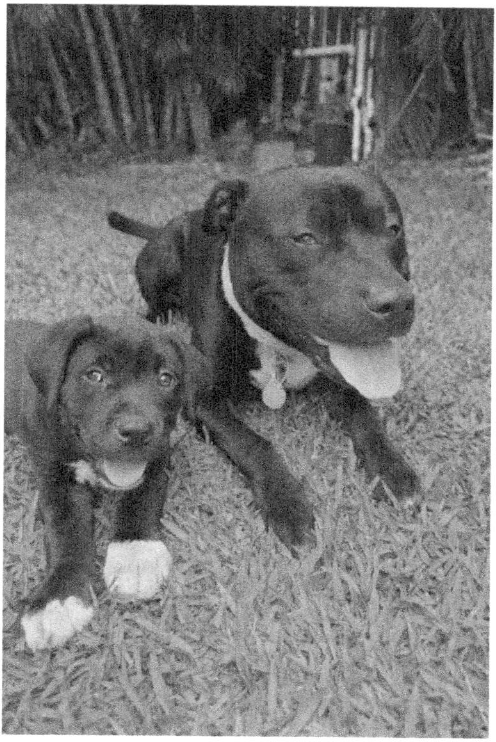

Why This Story Matters

Before there was illness, before there were timelines, medications, or intensive care monitors, there was simply love.

There was Cher, small, determined, and learning the world with her whole body. There was Elton, steady, watchful, and patient in a way dogs seem uniquely able to sustain. And there was the quiet, ordinary miracle of sharing a life with them. The walks that anchor days. The routines that give shape to time. The way a home reorganises itself around the presence of dogs. The way they notice us, follow us, wait for us, and forgive us without condition.

Dogs do not simply live alongside us. They shape how we move through our days. They slow us when the world accelerates and pull us into the present when attention drifts elsewhere. They offer companionship without negotiation and loyalty without transaction. In return, they ask for little. Food. Safety. Care. And to be recognised as sentient beings whose inner lives matter.

Cher's story is not extraordinary because she survived tetanus. It is extraordinary because it reveals how much responsibility is carried inside love. Loving a dog is not only about affection or enjoyment. It is about stewardship. It is about choosing, repeatedly and deliberately, to show up for a being who cannot describe their pain, explain their needs, or argue for their future. Dogs rely on humans to notice when something is wrong. They rely on us to persist when explanations do not resolve. They rely on us to carry decision-making when their bodies cannot.

Elton's presence in this story matters as well. Not because he was ill, but because he adapted. He waited. He moderated his play. He became gentler without instruction. In doing so, he reflected something essential about dogs. They meet us where we are. They adjust to circumstances without resentment. They offer patience before we recognise our own need for it. Watching Elton make space for Cher underscored that healing is not only clinical. It is also relational. Recovery unfolds not just through medication and management, but through the safety created by steady companionship.

From here, the story widens. Not toward illness, but toward legacy. Toward the dogs who will come after Cher. Toward the lives that may be safer, longer, or less interrupted because someone noticed a small change and chose not to dismiss it. And toward Cher herself, not as a case study or survivor, but as a dog who returned to play, curiosity, and presence in the world.

This story matters not because tetanus is rare, frightening, or complex. It matters because dogs enrich human lives in ways that are immeasurable, and that enrichment carries obligation. Not the obligation of perfection or certainty, but the obligation of commitment. Commitment to attention. Commitment to persistence. Commitment to care that continues when reassurance is tempting but resolution has not yet arrived.

The chapters that follow are about what remains after crisis recedes. They explore the responsibilities that endure beyond acute illness and the ways love continues to act long after fear has passed. They recognise that guardianship does not peak during emergency. It deepens afterward, in the quieter work of protection, patience, and follow-through.

This story matters because love does not end when the emergency is over.

It becomes more deliberate.

Chapter 19

For the Puppies Who Come After

This chapter is not about Cher.

It begins with that statement deliberately, because Cher's story, while personal and specific, is not the destination. It is the entry point. What follows exists to translate the experience of one dog into something that can quietly shape outcomes for others. This chapter occupies the space beyond crisis, where experience becomes knowledge and knowledge becomes responsibility.

For the puppies who come after, the most important protection we can offer is not vigilance driven by fear, but familiarity built through presence. Fear sharpens attention only during crisis. Familiarity is cultivated long before anything appears wrong. It develops through living alongside a dog closely enough that their normal becomes instinctive. This kind of knowing is not anxious or hyper-alert. It is calm, embodied, and relational. It allows concern to arise without panic and curiosity to replace dismissal. When familiarity is present, care is guided by recognition rather than reaction.

Dogs do not communicate illness through words, and they rarely announce it in ways that demand immediate alarm. Instead, they communicate through posture, tone, rhythm, and subtle deviation from their own baseline. A shoulder that holds tension where it once softened. A face that no longer fully releases during sleep. A gait that appears effortful rather than playful. These are not symptoms in the conventional sense. They are shifts in expression and ease, in how a body occupies space. Dogs show us how they feel long before they can show us what is wrong, but only when someone is close enough to notice the difference.

That baseline is not learned through routine care alone. It is not established through feeding schedules, veterinary visits, or structured activity. It is learned through proximity and repetition. Through unremarkable moments accumulated over time. Through noticing how a dog breathes when asleep and how that breathing changes with age, exertion, or comfort. Through recognising how their face settles when they are truly relaxed, how their ears rest when nothing is being asked of them, and how their body moves when it is not compensating for strain. Baseline is built in quiet, ordinary hours when nothing appears to be happening and nothing needs to be fixed.

Without this reference point, early change has nowhere to register. A tired eye looks unremarkable. A stiff movement appears consistent with growth. A change in posture is explained as mood. Each sign remains isolated, plausible, and easily dismissed. With familiarity, those same changes carry meaning. They are not alarming on their own, but they are noticeable. They stand out not because they are dramatic, but because they are different. Familiarity allows the body to be understood as a whole rather than a collection of parts. It transforms small deviations into information rather than background noise.

With that depth of knowing in place, even subtle change matters. Not because it demands immediate action, but because it invites attention rather than dismissal. Familiarity creates the conditions for concern to arise without certainty and without fear. It allows an owner to say that something is new and to trust that assessment even when they cannot yet explain why. For the puppies who come after, this kind of presence is protective. It often marks the difference between early recognition and delayed response, between a pattern noticed in time and one only understood in hindsight.

Cher's early signs were not dramatic, and that is precisely why they mattered. There was no single moment that demanded urgency and no obvious marker that declared a medical emergency. What existed instead were small deviations that only became visible through comparison. Her body did not collapse or fail suddenly. It changed subtly. These changes did not ask for diagnosis. They asked for recognition. They required someone who knew what normal looked like well enough to see when it had shifted. In situations like this, expertise does not arrive first. Attention does. When attention is grounded in familiarity, it can become lifesaving.

For future puppies, this distinction is critical. Their safety depends less on an owner's medical knowledge than on their willingness to notice difference without immediately explaining it away. Growth spurts, weather changes, developmental phases, mood fluctuations, and personality variation are often reasonable explanations. Sometimes they are correct. The risk arises not in considering these explanations, but in using them to close inquiry rather than keep it open. When reassurance becomes reflexive rather than reflective, and when "probably nothing" ends the conversation instead of beginning it, early opportunity is lost. The ability to tolerate uncertainty rather than resolve it prematurely is one of the most protective skills an owner can develop.

This chapter also asks that illness be understood as a pattern that emerges over time rather than a single event that announces itself clearly. Noticing one change is rarely enough. A dog that drinks slightly more, sleeps less deeply, carries more tension, or tires more easily may still appear healthy by conventional measures. Each of these signs, in isolation, is survivable and often transient. It is their persistence, overlap, and evolution that matter. Pattern recognition requires patience. It asks the observer to remember yesterday, compare it to today, and remain engaged long enough to notice when the trend does not resolve.

Early illness rarely progresses in a straight line. Dogs may appear better one day and worse the next. They may compensate effectively for periods of time, masking underlying strain. Improvement can occur without recovery, and fluctuation can create false reassurance. This inconsistency is not evidence that concern is misplaced. It is often a feature of neurological and systemic illness itself. For the puppies who come after, safety lies in understanding that illness frequently announces itself quietly, inconsistently, and without urgency long before it becomes unmistakable. Waiting for clarity can mean waiting too long.

Recognising patterns is not about becoming fearful or hypervigilant. It is about allowing unresolved change to retain its meaning. It is about trusting familiarity to provide context when certainty is not yet available. When owners observe without rushing to explain, they create space for early intervention, second opinions, and continued assessment. Protection begins here, not with expertise, but with attention that remains engaged even when the story is incomplete.

Cher's diagnosis did not come from certainty. It came from persistence. From returning when reassurance failed to resolve concern. From declining to accept waiting when waiting produced more questions than answers. For future puppies, this reveals a difficult truth. Systems tend toward closure. Advocacy requires resisting that momentum when something remains unresolved. It does not challenge expertise. It supplements it with lived observation that cannot be replicated within a consultation room.

This chapter frames advocacy as a sustained role rather than a single moment of insistence. Advocacy is not confrontation or escalation alone. It is the quieter and more demanding work of remaining present when clarity is absent and progress is slow. Guardianship requires engagement across uncertainty, fatigue, and doubt, particularly when there is no clear endpoint. It means returning to conversations, asking questions again, and tolerating the emotional strain of not knowing whether today's effort will matter tomorrow. Advocacy exists in duration rather than intensity.

In practical terms, this commitment is unremarkable in appearance. It involves attending follow-up appointments even when nothing appears worse. It includes tracking small changes that never escalate dramatically but never fully resolve. It requires administering medication consistently, even when routines are disrupted and sleep is broken. It means noticing when improvement plateaus, when subtle regression appears, and when reassurance no longer matches reality. Advocacy is not loud or heroic. It is repetitive, procedural, and persistent.

Responsibility does not guarantee outcomes, and advocacy does not ensure recovery. It widens the margin in which recovery becomes possible.

This form of commitment is emotionally taxing because it offers little immediate reward. There is rarely affirmation that persistence is justified. Often, there is only the knowledge that disengaging would be easier and therefore risky. Sustained advocacy requires resisting the urge to normalise concern simply because it is inconvenient. It asks guardians to remain responsive even when others assume the crisis has passed and when the dog appears outwardly stable. Stability is not the same as resolution, and advocacy requires holding that distinction even when it becomes exhausting.

Preparation for future puppies matters long before illness appears. This is not preparation rooted in anticipation of catastrophe, but in understanding what guardianship entails when things do not resolve quickly. Veterinary care is rarely linear. It can be complex, prolonged, and costly. Recovery often transfers responsibility from clinic to home and from professionals to owners. Entering guardianship without acknowledging this reality leaves both dogs and humans vulnerable when the unexpected occurs.

Cher's survival was shaped not only by medical treatment, but by the structural protection of private pet insurance. At no point did financial limitation determine the course of action. Treatment decisions were driven by physiology, not affordability. Access to care created time. Time allowed investigation. Investigation allowed diagnosis. Diagnosis allowed recovery. Each step depended on the one before it. For many dogs, this chain breaks early not because recovery is impossible, but because resources are exhausted before clarity emerges. When care becomes conditional on affordability, advocacy is constrained and outcomes narrow.

Financial preparedness is not pessimism or indulgence. It is ethical infrastructure. It allows decisions to be made in the dog's best interest rather than under crisis conditions. Whether through insurance, savings, or planning, sustained access to care creates space for medicine to function as intended. Advocacy requires that space.

This chapter also addresses restraint, and the frequent misunderstanding of what care should look like during recovery. Healing is not intuitive. Human instinct seeks comfort, reassurance, and a rapid return to normal life. Survival feels like a reason to restore freedom. In complex neurological recovery, that instinct can be harmful. Cher's recovery required stillness rather than stimulation, boundaries rather than freedom, and management rather than spontaneity. Care was not about adding experiences back in. It was about holding them away.

Restraint is often mistaken for deprivation, particularly in young dogs whose developmental drive is exploration and play. In reality, restraint during recovery is protection. A nervous system that is healing lacks the capacity to regulate movement, excitement, and exertion safely. Signals that normally govern recovery and inhibition remain unstable. Allowing freedom too early increases risk rather than strength. For future puppies, love may require saying no to joy in order to preserve healing. Recovery must not be equated with normalcy.

This restraint is emotionally difficult because it contradicts instinct. Watching a dog want to move, play, and participate while knowing they cannot safely do so creates a distinct form of distress. It requires overriding empathy-driven impulses in favour of outcome-driven decisions. Stillness is not passive. It is active containment. Boundaries are not punitive. They function as structural supports for a system that cannot yet support itself.

Recovery does not end at discharge. It relocates. Responsibility shifts from teams of professionals to individual households. Care continues without monitors, rotating staff, or built-in environmental controls. Toileting requires planning rather than convenience. Hydration requires supervision. Movement becomes calculated rather than spontaneous. Medication schedules become fixed and unforgiving. Precision matters even as fatigue accumulates. This labour continues quietly while the rest of life proceeds around it.

For the puppies who come after, this chapter makes explicit what is often left unsaid. Recovery is labour. It is sustained effort without immediate feedback. It is physically demanding, emotionally draining, and frequently isolating. It requires patience not only with the dog, but with oneself. Outcomes are secured not in dramatic moments, but in ordinary days where routines are maintained, restraint is held, and care is delivered without witness.

Recovery happens in the long aftermath, not the crisis. It unfolds through structure rather than freedom and through consistency rather than instinct.

Time in recovery is not measured in neat units or projected milestones. It is an open-ended commitment entered without certainty. Cher's nervous system healed according to biological processes that cannot be rushed or predicted. Improvement did not arrive steadily. It appeared briefly, stalled, and returned in altered form. Progress emerged in fragments rather than phases.

Periods of apparent stagnation were common. These plateaus were psychologically harder than setbacks, because they offered no feedback at all. What appeared as stillness was often silent repair. The nervous system recalibrates internally long before outward function stabilises.

For future puppies, expectations must be honest. Recovery does not move predictably. It does not reward effort with immediate results. It fluctuates. This variability is not failure. It is adjustment.

The central task is not acceleration, but presence. Presence requires endurance without narrative and consistency without guarantee. It means holding boundaries even when improvement tempts relaxation and continuing care when motivation fades. Time is not something to pass through. It is something to inhabit.

Recovery is not about reaching a finish line. It is about remaining committed long enough for the body to find its way back on its own terms.

The emotional cost of this commitment is substantial and rarely acknowledged. Caregiving becomes a sustained state of vigilance that does not pause. Fear of regression, fear of missing subtle change, and fear of undoing progress accompany every decision. This strain spills outward into households and relationships. Other dogs adapt, wait, and adjust. Guilt accumulates. Attention is redistributed. There is no perfect balance, only the best possible one under constraint.

This labour remains largely invisible. There is no recognition for restraint or vigilance. The work occurs in quiet spaces, controlled routines, delayed pleasures, and postponed normality. Life continues alongside it. Recovery overlays rather than replaces daily responsibility.

For future guardians, acknowledging this cost matters. Not to discourage care, but to normalise the weight of it. Feeling overwhelmed does not indicate failure. It reflects sustained engagement. Guilt signals care stretched across multiple lives, not misallocation. Grief for what is temporarily lost can coexist with commitment to healing.

Love does not make this work easy. It makes it necessary.

This chapter ultimately concerns legacy, though not a chosen one. Cher did not choose to become a reference point. She simply became unwell and then survived. Through that survival, something now carries forward. Her experience becomes a marker for attention. A reminder that early change matters even when it resists explanation. That survival may depend less on brilliance or speed than on persistence and proximity.

This is not a chapter about fear. Fear narrows and demands certainty. Fear seeks resolution or retreat. What carried Cher through was steadier than fear.

It was responsibility carried with tenderness.

Tenderness does not mean softness. It means staying close without force, holding boundaries without anger, and remaining attentive without panic. Responsibility carried this way is quiet and repetitive. It shows up in how a dog is watched while sleeping, how change is noted before it is named, and how care continues when reassurance does not arrive.

For the puppies who come after, survival often begins before crisis appears. It begins with familiarity built through presence. With knowing how a dog moves on an ordinary day and how their face settles when relaxed. Without this baseline, early change has nowhere to land. With it, even subtle deviation becomes legible.

Survival also begins with persistence, preparation, and the capacity to remain present when clarity is slow. It begins with understanding that veterinary care may be complex, prolonged, and costly. That recovery often shifts responsibility home. That restraint may be required long after visible danger has passed.

This chapter does not exist to warn. It exists to witness. In that witnessing, it quietly widens the margin of safety for the puppies who come after.

Chapter 20

Cher Today

Cher today is not a symbol. She is five and a half months old.

That detail matters because age anchors recovery in reality rather than abstraction. At five and a half months, she is still a puppy whose body and nervous system are actively developing. She is still learning how to inhabit the world, how to regulate herself within it, and how to grow into the dog she is becoming. Recovery at this stage does not mean returning to a finished state. It means resuming development where it was interrupted.

She now weighs thirty kilograms. This weight does not reflect excess or urgency. It reflects strength and proportionate growth returning on schedule. Her body has filled out naturally, without strain or compensatory tension. Where her system once worked to manage instability, it now grows with ease. Muscle tone has normalised, movement flows without effort, and physical development has re-entered a stable trajectory.

Her coat provides another quiet indicator of systemic health. It is thick, dense, and glossy, lying smoothly along her body and warm under the hand. The dullness that often accompanies prolonged stress or metabolic strain is absent. This change is not cosmetic. Skin and coat are among the last systems to fully recover after significant physiological disruption. Their condition reflects internal stability rather than surface appearance. In Cher's case, it confirms what behaviour and movement already suggest. Her body is no longer operating in survival mode. It has shifted into growth.

Her eyes no longer carry the constant tension that once defined them. They rest fully when she sleeps. They soften when she is calm. They brighten with play, curiosity, and recognition. Expression has returned without vigilance or effort. This change is subtle, but it is significant, because neurological strain often shows itself first in the eyes and is among the last places where true release appears.

Her relationship with Elton has returned to balance. Their bond is playful, affectionate, and reciprocal. She seeks him out not from dependence, but from enjoyment. They wrestle, chase, rest together, and move through shared space with ease. Where interaction once required careful management and protection, it now unfolds naturally. Elton no longer moderates himself out of necessity, and Cher no longer requires shielding. With their equilibrium restored, the rhythm of the household has settled as well.

Play has returned in a regulated form. Cher runs because she can. She tumbles because it feels good. She rests when she is tired, not because her body demands it, but because she chooses to pause. This capacity for choice is one of the clearest indicators of neurological recovery. Her nervous system no longer overrides behaviour. Regulation has replaced compulsion, allowing body and intention to work together again.

She continues to learn quickly. She watches closely, absorbs cues, and responds with confidence rather than hesitation. Training is not a struggle or a task. It functions as a conversation grounded in trust. The foundations established before her illness were not erased. They were paused. When recovery allowed learning to resume, those foundations held. Early training built on clarity and consistency does not disappear during illness. It waits, and then it returns.

Cher thrives outdoors. She enjoys space, movement, and the presence of other dogs. Doggy daycare is no longer a milestone or test. It is a place of enjoyment. She plays with confidence, disengages when needed, and rests without prompting. What stands out is not her energy, but her regulation. She recognises her own limits and responds to them. These skills cannot be taught directly. They emerge when a nervous system is stable enough to support them.

Hydrotherapy remains part of her routine, but its role has changed. Weekly sessions at K9 Aquatics Coomera, are no longer scheduled just for treatment they have started to return to pleasure. She enters the water eagerly, moving with strength and coordination. What was once a carefully controlled rehabilitation environment has become a place of enjoyment. Rick observes her with the calm assurance of someone who understands recovery as a state rather than a checklist. He sees a dog whose body has returned to itself, knowing that she can relapse at any time. All care is taken during these sessions.

Cher shows no fear of veterinary care. She greets the clinic with familiarity and enthusiasm. Dr Siobhan is met with unrestrained affection, often requiring Cher to be settled before examination can proceed. This response reflects how her care was delivered during illness. The absence of force, the presence of consistency, and the respect shown for her limits preserved trust rather than eroding it. That trust remains intact.

Even now, care has not shifted into assumption. Monitoring continues. Recovery does not remove responsibility, and visible wellness does not mean the work is finished. There are evenings when small deviations still appear. A night where her eyes look bloodshot. A moment where her baseline expression is not quite equal. These are not emergencies, but they are cues. When they appear, activity is reduced without hesitation. Bed rest replaces stimulation. Stillness replaces movement. This is not regression. It is respect for the central nervous system, which heals and recalibrates in ways that cannot be observed directly. Muscles, posture, and behaviour may look resolved, while neurological load fluctuates quietly beneath the surface. Because the nervous system is invisible, care must remain observational rather than assumptive. Recovery continues not through optimism, but through attention to subtle signals and the willingness to respond conservatively when something does not fully align.

Tetanus recovery is not linear. Cher continues to experience relapses. They are not dramatic collapses, nor are they failures of care. They are part of the nature of tetanus when it has affected a developing nervous system. At five and a half months, she is still growing rapidly. Every growth spurt places new demand on the central nervous system. Neural pathways recalibrate. Muscles lengthen. Coordination shifts. During these periods, old vulnerability can resurface. Tension returns more quickly. Fatigue appears without obvious cause. Her baseline tightens in ways that are subtle but familiar.

When this happens, the response is immediate and conservative. Crate isolation resumes. Stimulation is reduced. Antibiotics are reintroduced at the first sign of potential bacterial exposure. A minor scrape that would be insignificant for most dogs becomes a veterinary consultation and preventative treatment. The vet remains on call. Monitoring intensifies. This is not overreaction. It is recognition that until the central nervous system has fully stabilised, small insults can carry disproportionate impact. Relapse does not mean she is failing. It means the healing process is still underway.

There are moments, during these cycles, when I question myself. I examine routines. I reconsider decisions. I wonder whether I missed something, allowed too much stimulation, misread a signal. That questioning is natural. But the pattern is consistent. Growth precedes vulnerability. Vulnerability precedes recalibration. Each relapse has resolved with the same disciplined return to stillness. What feels personal is in fact physiological.

Cher is currently living through one of these relapses.

And yet, even within it, the broader trajectory remains intact. Each cycle has shortened. Each recovery has been steadier. The central nervous system heals in increments, not declarations. What once required hospitalisation now requires vigilance at home. What once overwhelmed her system now resolves with early intervention and rest.

Cher does not remember being ill. She carries no narrative of fragility or fear. She lives forward, embodied in the present. Animals do not rehearse survival. They inhabit it. She knows only that she is alive, secure, and free to move through the world.

It would be easy to frame her as a symbol or a metaphor. That framing would be inaccurate.

Cher is evidence.

She demonstrates what early attention makes possible. She reflects what foundational training preserves. She shows what restraint, patience, and sustained care can return. Her development was interrupted, not erased. Her future was protected rather than rushed.

Cher today is not defined by what happened to her. She is defined by what was allowed to continue.

She has returned to the life she was always meant to live, even as that life occasionally requires renewed caution. She lives not as an example or a lesson, but as herself. She is not simply a dog in recovery. She is my dog, and she is a central part of my family. She belongs within the daily rhythms, shared responsibilities, and quiet attachments that shape a life lived together. Recovery did not return her to abstraction. It returned her to belonging.

This book may end here, but Cher's life does not. Her story is not closing. It is opening. What lies ahead for her is not defined by illness, but by growth, experience, and the ordinary, extraordinary continuity of a life still unfolding.

Cher's photos

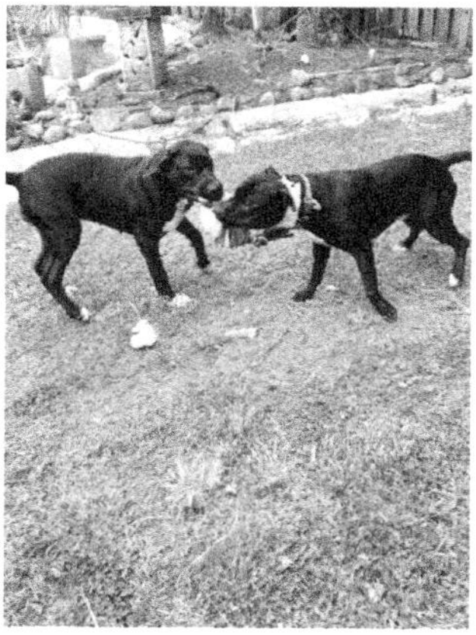

Playing with Elton

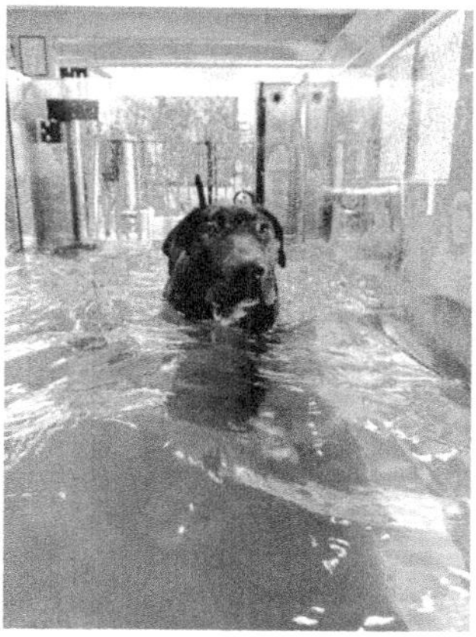

Enjoying Hydrotherapy

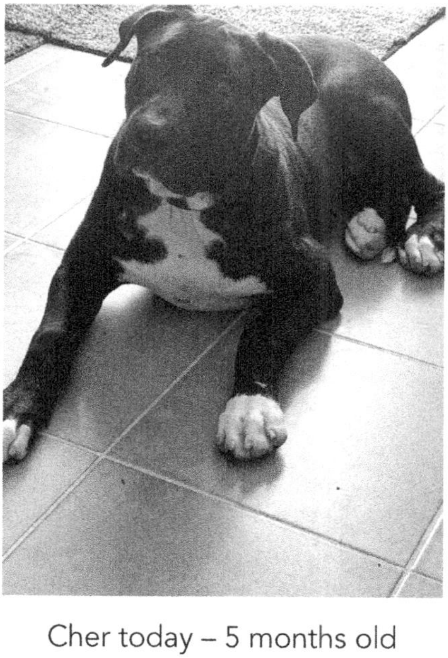

Cher today – 5 months old

GLOSSARY

Plain Language Guide for Pet Owners

Why This Glossary Exists

Veterinary ICU and tetanus involve complex terminology that can overwhelm owners during already stressful moments. Understanding these terms does not change the outcome, but it can change how supported, informed, and grounded an owner feels while navigating care.

Knowledge does not replace trust.

But it can sit alongside it.

ICU Related Terms

ICU (Intensive Care Unit)

A level of veterinary care where animals are monitored continuously and supported when their bodies cannot safely manage on their own. ICU focuses on stabilisation, monitoring, and preventing complications rather than rapid cures.

Critical Care

Care provided to patients whose condition is life threatening or unstable and requires constant observation and rapid intervention.

Monitoring

Ongoing observation of vital signs such as breathing, heart rate, muscle tone, oxygen levels, and responsiveness. Monitoring allows staff to detect small changes before they become emergencies.

Sedation

Medication used to calm the nervous system, reduce muscle tension, and prevent distress or spasms. Sedation is carefully adjusted to keep the patient comfortable without suppressing breathing or protective reflexes.

Low Stimulus Environment
A controlled setting with minimal noise, light, touch, and movement. In tetanus cases, stimulation can trigger painful muscle spasms, so calm is a critical part of treatment.

Supportive Care
Treatment that supports the body while it heals rather than curing the disease directly. This can include fluids, nutrition, temperature control, oxygen, pain relief, and comfort measures.

Fluid Therapy
Intravenous fluids used to maintain hydration, support circulation, and prevent complications when a dog cannot drink normally.

Nutritional Support

Methods used to ensure a dog receives adequate nutrition when eating or swallowing is unsafe or difficult. This may include assisted feeding or specialised diets.

Aspiration

When food, liquid, or saliva enters the airway instead of the stomach. This can lead to pneumonia and is a serious risk in dogs with swallowing difficulties.

Vital Signs

Basic measurements such as heart rate, breathing rate, temperature, and oxygen saturation that indicate how well the body is functioning.

Stability

A state where the dog's condition is not worsening, even if it is not yet improving. In ICU, stability is often the primary goal.

Titration

The gradual adjustment of medication doses based on the dog's response. Titration helps balance effectiveness with safety.

Neurological Monitoring

Assessment of reflexes, posture, muscle tone, and responsiveness to track changes in nervous system function over time.

Complications

Secondary problems that can arise during illness or treatment, such as breathing difficulties, infections, or nutritional issues.

Tetanus Related Terms

Tetanus

A neurological disease caused by a toxin produced by the bacterium *Clostridium tetani*. It leads to sustained muscle contraction, stiffness, and rigidity.

Clostridium tetani

A spore forming bacterium found in soil, dust, and animal faeces. The bacteria itself does not spread widely in the body, but produces a powerful toxin at the site of infection.

Tetanospasmin

The neurotoxin produced by *Clostridium tetani*. It interferes with the nervous system's ability to signal muscles to relax.

Anaerobic

An organism that thrives in low oxygen environments. *Clostridium tetani* becomes active when oxygen levels beneath the skin are low.

Spore

A dormant, highly resilient form of bacteria that can survive harsh environmental conditions for long periods.

Neurotoxin

A toxin that affects the nervous system. In tetanus, the neurotoxin disrupts communication between nerves and muscles.

Retrograde Nerve Transport

The process by which the tetanus toxin travels along nerves toward the spinal cord and brain rather than through the bloodstream.

Muscle Rigidity

Persistent muscle contraction that prevents normal movement and relaxation. This is a hallmark of tetanus.

Spasm

Sudden, involuntary muscle contractions that can be triggered by noise, touch, light, or movement in tetanus patients.

Lockjaw

Stiffness of the jaw muscles that can make opening the mouth difficult. This can interfere with eating and swallowing.

Swallow Reflex

The coordinated muscle response that allows safe swallowing. In tetanus, this reflex can be impaired, increasing the risk of aspiration.

Incubation Period

The time between bacterial entry and the appearance of symptoms. In tetanus, this can range from days to weeks.

Clinical Diagnosis

A diagnosis based on observed signs, progression, and exclusion of other conditions rather than a single definitive test.

Antitoxin

A medication that neutralises tetanus toxin circulating in the body. It does not reverse toxin already bound to nerves but can prevent further progression.

Resistance vs Immunity

Resistance means a species is less likely to develop disease. Immunity means protection from disease. Dogs are more resistant to tetanus than humans but are not immune.

Recovery Phase

The prolonged period during which nerves slowly regain function and muscles gradually relax. Recovery from tetanus can take weeks to months.

Growth, Nutrition, and Development During Tetanus Recovery

Growth Spurt (Puppy Development)

A normal developmental phase in young dogs marked by rapid increases in body size, muscle mass, and metabolic demand. Growth spurts significantly increase nutritional requirements and hunger signals, even when medical conditions restrict normal feeding.

Developmental Nutritional Demand

The increased need for calories, protein, and micronutrients during periods of rapid growth. In puppies recovering from tetanus, this demand may intensify frustration and hunger while safe feeding must remain slow and limited.

Restricted Feeding During Growth

A medically necessary limitation on food volume or delivery despite heightened hunger and developmental need. In tetanus recovery, restricted feeding protects swallowing safety and prevents aspiration, even when the body is actively demanding nourishment.

Controlled Nutritional Delivery

The deliberate provision of food in carefully measured amounts to meet essential needs without exceeding what the body can safely tolerate. This approach prioritises safety over satiety and is often required during neurological recovery.

Hunger Without Satiety

A state in which a dog experiences strong hunger signals but cannot achieve normal oral feeding satisfaction due to medical restrictions or tube feeding. This can increase distress, food focus, and behavioural challenges such as resource guarding.

Developmental Frustration

A predictable emotional and behavioural response seen in young animals whose normal growth driven behaviours, such as eating freely or playing, are restricted due to illness. This response is not pathological and resolves as recovery allows normal development to resume.

Veterinary Literature Referenced

Plain-Language Guide with APA References

This reference list exists to support understanding, not to replace veterinary care. It reflects the complexity of tetanus, recovery, and caregiving, and acknowledges that behind every clinical term is a lived experience shared between an animal and the human who chose to stay.

1. Canine Tetanus: Disease Mechanism and Clinical Presentation

These sources explain how tetanus develops in dogs, why they are considered more resistant than humans but not immune, and why early signs are often subtle, neurological, and easily misattributed. They support descriptions of muscle rigidity, spasms, lockjaw, swallowing impairment, and delayed diagnosis.

APA references:

- Greene, C. E. (2012). Infectious diseases of the dog and cat (4th ed.). Elsevier Saunders.
- Merck Veterinary Manual. (2023). Tetanus in dogs. Merck & Co.
- Boothe, D. M. (2015). Small animal clinical pharmacology and therapeutics (2nd ed.). Elsevier.

2. Tetanospasmin, Neurotoxicity, and Retrograde Nerve Transport

These references support explanations of how tetanus toxin travels along nerves rather than through the bloodstream, why antitoxin cannot reverse already-bound toxin, and why recovery depends on slow regeneration of nerve function.

APA references:

- Cook, T. M., Protheroe, R. T., & Handel, J. M. (2001). Tetanus: A review of the literature. *British Journal of Anaesthesia*, 87(3), 477–487.
- Uzal, F. A., & Songer, J. G. (2008). Diagnosis of Clostridium tetani infection in animals. *Journal of Veterinary Diagnostic Investigation*, 20(4), 447–452.

3. ICU Care, Critical Care, and Neurological Monitoring

These sources underpin the ICU glossary, including continuous monitoring, neurological assessment, titration of medications, stability versus improvement, and prevention of complications during prolonged hospitalisation.

APA references:

- Silverstein, D. C., & Hopper, K. (2015). *Small animal critical care medicine* (2nd ed.). Elsevier.
- Platt, S. R., & Olby, N. J. (2013). *BSAVA manual of canine and feline neurology* (4th ed.). BSAVA.

4. Sedation, Low-Stimulus Environments, and Spasm Prevention

These references support the need for sedation, environmental control, and minimal stimulation in tetanus patients, including why noise, light, and touch can provoke spasms.

APA references:

- Mathews, K. A. (2008). Pain management and sedation in critical patients. *Veterinary Clinics of North America: Small Animal Practice*, 38(6), 1289–1312.
- Taylor, P. M., & Robertson, S. A. (2004). Pain management in dogs and cats. *Journal of Small Animal Practice*, 45(2), 97–104.

5. Aspiration Risk and Swallowing Dysfunction

These sources support discussion of aspiration pneumonia risk, impaired swallow reflex, assisted feeding, and the necessity of controlled hydration and nutrition.

APA references:

- Ettinger, S. J., Feldman, E. C., & Côté, E. (2017). *Textbook of veterinary internal medicine* (8th ed.). Elsevier.
- Marks, S. L. (2011). Disorders of swallowing and aspiration risk in dogs. *Veterinary Clinics of North America: Small Animal Practice*, 41(2), 311–328.

6. Recovery Phase and Central Nervous System Healing

These references support the assertion that recovery is prolonged, nonlinear, and dependent on nervous system recalibration rather than simple muscle strength or symptom resolution.

APA references:

- de Lahunta, A., Glass, E., & Kent, M. (2015). *Veterinary neuroanatomy and clinical neurology* (4th ed.). Elsevier.
- Platt, S. R. (2009). Neurologic recovery and rehabilitation in dogs. *Veterinary Clinics of North America: Small Animal Practice*, 39(1), 1–21.

7. Home-Based Recovery and Owner-Delivered Care

These sources support the transition of care from hospital to home, including medication adherence, controlled movement, toileting on lead, and the owner's role in preventing regression.

APA references:

- Hopper, K., & Epstein, S. E. (2014). Caregiver roles in prolonged veterinary recovery. *Journal of Veterinary Emergency and Critical Care*, 24(4), 389–398.
- Overall, K. L. (2013). Manual of clinical behavioral medicine for dogs and cats. Elsevier.

8. Puppy Growth, Nutrition, and Increased Metabolic Demand

These references support the sections on growth spurts, heightened hunger, developmental nutritional demand, and the physiological conflict between growth needs and medically restricted feeding.

APA references:

- Case, L. P., Daristotle, L., Hayek, M. G., & Raasch, M. F. (2011). *Canine and feline nutrition* (3rd ed.). Elsevier Mosby.
- Hand, M. S., Thatcher, C. D., Remillard, R. L., Roudebush, P., & Novotny, B. J. (2010). *Small animal clinical nutrition*(5th ed.). Mark Morris Institute.

9. Restricted Feeding, Hunger Without Satiety, and Behavioural Effects

These sources support explanations of hunger without satiety, food fixation, frustration, and behavioural changes during prolonged feeding restriction.

APA references:

- Landsberg, G., Hunthausen, W., & Ackerman, L. (2013). *Behavior problems of the dog and cat* (3rd ed.). Saunders.
- Overall, K. L., & Love, M. (2001). Dog bites to humans: Demography, epidemiology, injury, and risk. *Journal of the American Veterinary Medical Association*, 218(12), 1923–1934.

10. Developmental Frustration and Behavioural Resilience

These references underpin the concept of developmental frustration in young dogs whose normal growth behaviours are restricted, and why this is adaptive rather than pathological.

APA references:

- Scott, J. P., & Fuller, J. L. (1965). *Genetics and the social behaviour of the dog*. University of Chicago Press.
- Serpell, J. A., & Jagoe, J. A. (1995). Early experience and the development of behaviour. *The Domestic Dog*. Cambridge University Press.

11. Emotional Toll of Caregiving and Multi-Pet Households

These sources support the emotional strain on caregivers, redistribution of attention among pets, guilt, fatigue, and the psychological burden of prolonged responsibility.

APA references:

- Kogan, L. R., Schoenfeld-Tacher, R., & Hellyer, P. W. (2018). Veterinary caregivers and emotional labour. *Journal of Veterinary Medical Education*, 45(2), 169–176.
- Rollin, B. E. (2006). *An introduction to veterinary medical ethics*. Blackwell Publishing.

12. Prognosis, Mortality, and Ethical Decision-Making

These references support statements that not all dogs survive tetanus, outcomes vary widely, and access to care strongly influences prognosis.

APA references:

- Bandt, C., & Rozanski, E. A. (2014). Tetanus in dogs: A retrospective study. *Journal of Veterinary Emergency and Critical Care*, 24(5), 502–509.
- Merck Veterinary Manual. (2023). *Prognosis and outcomes in canine tetanus.* Merck & Co.

About the Author

Julie Dimmick is a best-selling author, executive leader, and values-based strategist whose work sits at the intersection of policy, performance, people, and responsibility.

Her writing and leadership are shaped by a career spent navigating complex systems under pressure, where decisions carry real human consequences and outcomes are rarely tidy. Across public and private sectors, Julie has led multi-million-dollar transformation programs, overseen regulatory and governance reform, and guided organisations through periods of high-stakes change. She is sought out when clarity is required, complexity cannot be avoided, and accountability matters.

Julie's most recent book, *Hot Flush, Cold Truth: Beyond the Pause. Women, Work, and Policy Reform*, is both deeply personal and structurally rigorous. It combines lived experience, executive insight, and systemic critique to expose how menopause has been silenced, misdiagnosed, and dismissed, and how it can be reclaimed as a catalyst for health, equity, and reform.

She is also the author of the best-selling *The Trump Effect: What One Man Reveals About How the World Evolves*, a ground-breaking analysis of leadership, power, and culture through the lens of Spiral Dynamics. That work established Julie as a thought leader in values-based analysis, bridging psychology, politics, and global systems to explore how individual behaviour reflects and shapes collective evolution.

Julie is the creator of ValCoRE™ (Values, Consciousness, Resilience, and Evolution), a leadership and organisational framework designed to help individuals and institutions understand power, navigate complexity, and lead without losing themselves. ValCoRE™ has been applied across corporate transformation, executive coaching, and personal development, supporting leaders to act with integrity in environments that reward speed over reflection.

Animal stewardship is not separate from this work. It is an extension of it.

Julie approaches guardianship with the same principles that guide her leadership: attention, responsibility, persistence, and ethical care in the absence of certainty. Her experience advocating for a critically ill puppy reinforced a truth that runs through all her work, that systems do not protect what they do not see, and outcomes are shaped not only by expertise, but by sustained presence and willingness to remain engaged when answers are slow to arrive.

At the core of Julie's writing is a commitment to giving voice where silence is costly, whether that silence exists in workplaces, institutions, or the quiet early signs of vulnerability in those who cannot speak for themselves. Through her books, speaking, and advisory work, she champions a model of leadership and stewardship rooted not in control or certainty, but in responsibility carried with clarity, empathy, and resolve.

Made in the USA
Monee, IL
05 November 2026

67808951R00167